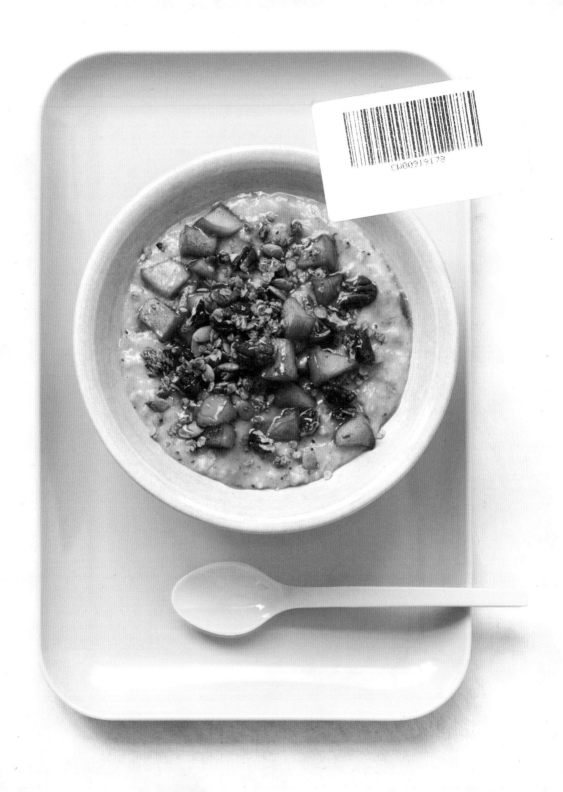

# the new
# PORRIDGE

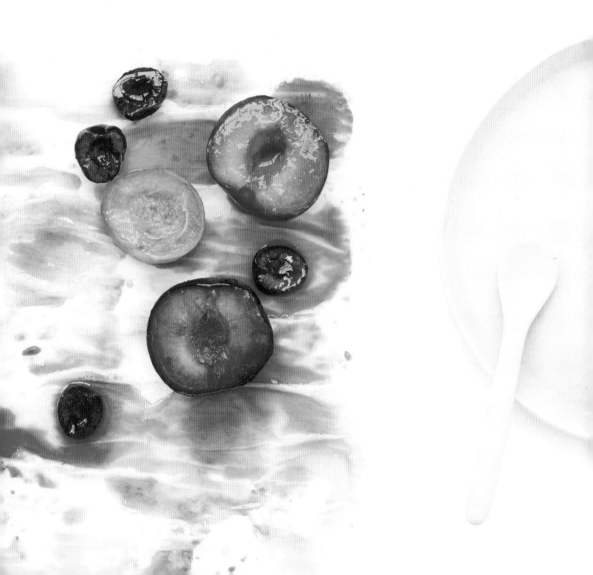

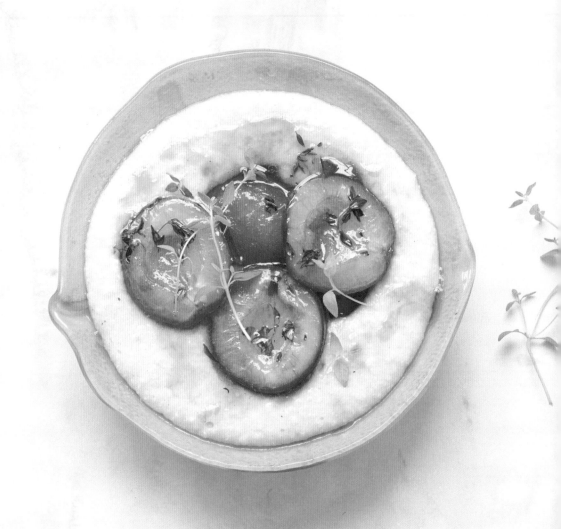

# the new
# PORRIDGE

## GRAIN-BASED NUTRITION BOWLS FOR MORNING, NOON AND NIGHT

LEAH VANDERVELDT

PHOTOGRAPHY BY
CLARE WINFIELD

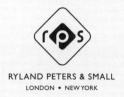

RYLAND PETERS & SMALL
LONDON • NEW YORK

**Senior Designer** Sonya Nathoo
**Commissioning Editor** Alice
Sambrook
**Text Editors** Kate Reeves-Brown
and Emily Preece-Morrison
**Production** Mai-Ling Collyer
**Editorial Director** Julia Charles
**Art Director** Leslie Harrington
**Publisher** Cindy Richards

**Food Stylist** Emily Kydd
**Prop Stylist** Alexander Breeze
**Indexer** Vanessa Bird

First published in 2018
by Ryland Peters & Small
20–21 Jockey's Fields
London WC1R 4BW and
341 E 116th Street, New York, 10029
www.rylandpeters.com
10 9 8 7 6 5 4 3 2 1

ISBN: 978-1-84975-930-4

A CIP record for this book is
available from the British Library.
US Library of Congress CIP data has
been applied for.

Printed in China

**Notes**
• Both British (Metric) and American
(Imperial and US cups)
measurements are included in these
recipes for your convenience,
however it is important to work with
one set of measurements and not
alternate between the two.
• Buy unwaxed citrus fruit and wash
before zesting. If you can only find
treated fruit, scrub well before using.
• If using edible flowers, make sure
they are food-safe.

**DEDICATION**

For the people who want
to be 'morning people'.

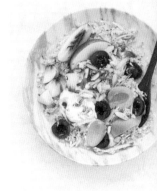

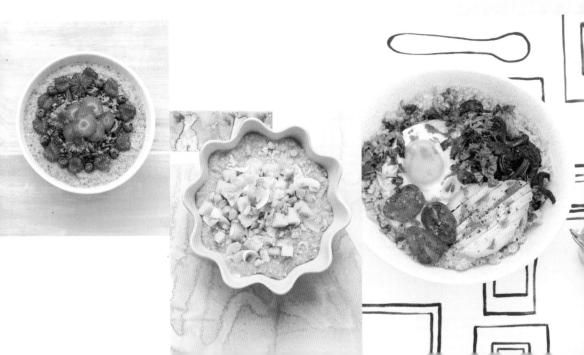

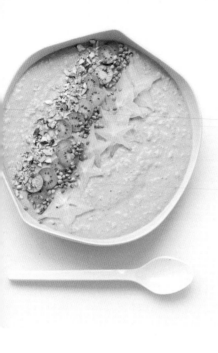

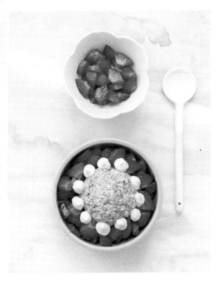

# CONTENTS

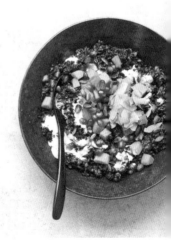

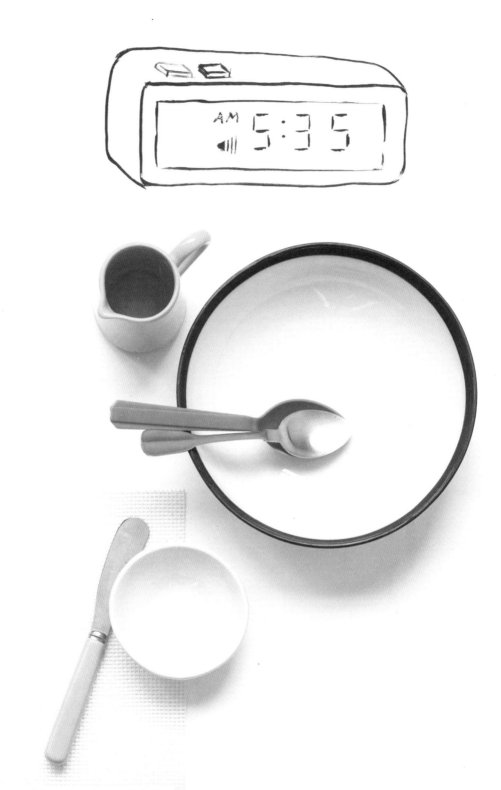

# INTRODUCTION

Mornings have always been a struggle for me. For as long as I can remember I've been a snooze button-hitting, grumpy, slow-paced, decidedly non-morning person. I was also never really a breakfast person, especially in my late teens and early 20s. When I decided to give running in the morning a try, I realized that my body needed fuel very shortly after my a.m. jog around the park. With a few missteps along the way, I started coming up with nourishing, balanced breakfasts to keep me going, and once breakfast was reinstated as a part of my routine, I've never looked back.

Since then, porridge has been a beloved go-to meal for me. I use the word porridge (instead of the American oatmeal) to describe these breakfasts because they go way beyond oats – in fact, you can make pretty much any grain or even non-grain into a porridge. When it occurred to me that I can change up flavours in the form of new grains, toppings and healthy fats on a whim, I was hooked. With its versatility and cosy factor, it's now the base I most often reach for. I even fell in love with its cold cousins, overnight oats and bircher muesli, for when the weather doesn't warrant a warm bowl of anything. I learned that porridge doesn't even have to be a morning meal, savoury versions are great for lunch or dinner.

One of the best things about porridge to me is that I can either make it ahead or use quick-cooking grains, such as rolled/old-fashioned oats, to throw breakfast together without much thought in the mornings. Knowing I'm a few minutes away from a hearty, filling and delicious breakfast helps me launch out of bed, even on those cold, grey winter mornings.

Porridge is a great start to the day for a few reasons, but especially for its inherently high fibre content. When combined with fat and protein, this formula can help you get through the toughest of mornings.

The benefits of my breakfast habit go beyond the simple pleasures of a good meal, too. Once I started eating breakfast regularly, I noticed a shift in my productivity and actually found that my sharpest and most motivating time for getting things done (and done right) was the morning. Without porridge to motivate me, it would have taken me a very long time to realize this. But now I leverage this productive and high-energy time in my day to tackle the most challenging aspects of my work. And, as silly as it might sound, I kind of owe it all to porridge.

I hope the recipes in this book help make your day a little cosier and happier.

# THE BASICS OF MAKING PORRIDGE

MAKING PORRIDGE IS ALL ABOUT PERSONAL PREFERENCE, BUT
THESE ARE THE MAIN AREAS I FOCUS ON THAT WILL HELP YOU TO
COOK A PORRIDGE THAT'S JUST RIGHT FOR YOU.

## SOAKING

While I realize that soaking your grains (whether you're using oats, quinoa or farro) can be a bit of a hassle, it's actually very helpful for two main reasons. Firstly, the longer you soak your grains (overnight is great!), the quicker they will cook. As grains are dried, soaking rehydrates them, and starts the cooking process early without any heat. Secondly, grains contain phytic acid. This protects the grains in nature, but can sometimes be rough on our digestive systems. To significantly reduce the phytic acid in your grains, you can soak them with a spritz of lemon juice or a small splash of neutral vinegar – you won't taste it, because you'll rinse this off before you cook the grains. The acid helps break down those protective compounds on the grain, making it easier on your body.

If you can't soak grains overnight, even just a bit of time is great. All you have to do is cover them generously with water and add a splash of acid, then drain and rinse when you're ready to use. In the recipes which include longer-cooking grains, I remind you to soak them before using, but you can do it for all grains if you like. Don't worry though, if you just don't have the time and skip the soaking step, it's not the end of the world.

## SWEETNESS

The level of sweetness in any of these recipes is always adjustable. I tend to err on the side of less sweet, so you can always add more maple syrup, honey, dates, bananas, etc., if you like.

I do think cold or overnight oats and puddings need a little extra sweetness to taste amazing, so I've kept that in mind for the cold chapter.

## SEASONING

All grains are pretty bland if they are not seasoned properly. Trust me, even the sweetest of porridges can benefit from a pinch or so of salt – it brings out the natural flavours of whatever grains, spices and flavours you're using.

Fresh lemon juice is also a powerful seasoning tool. I find that when things are feeling a little too stodgy, sweet or one-note, a little spritz of lemon perks everything up ever so slightly, without being overpowering.

## COOKING TIMES

The length of cooking times varies according to the type of grains you have, for example, if they're pearled, partially pearled or hulled; if you've soaked them and for how long. These factors can all give you slightly different results than the recipe suggests. If something is looking extra soupy, you might need to cook it uncovered for another 10–15 minutes. Conversely, if your grains have absorbed all of the liquid quickly, leaving it less porridge-y than you'd like, add some more water or milk. Know what your preference is, and let that guide you.

## REHEATING

I'm all about making a batch of porridge ahead of time and reheating it throughout the week – especially for recipes with longer cooking times. Keep in mind that most grains continue to absorb liquid as they cool, so many porridges will require a little extra liquid combined with a gentle heat, instead of being blasted in the microwave. For the best results, put your cold porridge, along with a small splash of liquid (water or milk), into a saucepan, then bring up to a simmer over a medium-low heat, stirring often. Once it's heated through, assess the texture and see if you need more liquid, then serve as you would normally.

## LIQUID AMOUNTS

I state liquid amounts for all of the porridges, but ultimately it's about personal preference (and the specific grains you have, and whether you've soaked them or not). I tried to use liquid amounts to create porridges that are not overly soupy or stodgy, but you might require more or less to get them to your desired consistency. See what you like and adjust accordingly.

## CHANGE IT UP

If you don't have barley, sub it for brown rice or coarse oatmeal/steel-cut oats. Work with what you have and adjust these recipes to your taste. Perhaps you'd prefer a certain topping combo with a different grain base to what's listed – mix and match, my friend!

# GRAIN TALK

FOR THIS BOOK, I MOSTLY USED THE WHOLE FORM OF GRAINS, AS
THOSE WERE THE EASIEST TO FIND IN MY PART OF THE WORLD. PEARL
BARLEY AND OATS (WHICH ARE EITHER CUT OR STEAMED AND ROLLED
FLAT) ARE THE EXCEPTION.

Whatever you have the easiest access to
(and what you like best) are the best kind
of grains you can use. Cracked or rolled
versions of grains are great for porridges, if
you can find them. I actually had a hard time
buying many of these in a pinch (although
the internet is always helpful for that sort of
thing!). But if you can find the rolled version
such as quinoa or barley flakes, or the
cracked version such as cream of buckwheat
cereal, these will all play well in most
recipes, and your cooking times will
decrease. Just make sure the only ingredient
in your buckwheat 'cereal', as it's often
called, is the grain itself.

## COARSE OATMEAL/STEEL CUT OATS
## AND ROLLED/OLD-FASHIONED OATS

Oats are naturally gluten-free, but they
are often processed in places where other
glutinous foods are processed, so it is
important to read labels carefully if you have
a serious allergy. Oats are loaded with
minerals like manganese, magnesium and
zinc, and important B vitamins, not to
mention fibre and protein. This porridge
grain helps reduce bad cholesterol levels
and prevents heart disease with its unique
profile of antioxidants. Plus, it's incredibly
versatile and a great base for any porridge.

## QUINOA

Quinoa, which is gluten-free, is actually a
pseudo-grain, meaning it's a seed that acts
like a grain. It's also a complete protein and
contains all the essential amino acids. There
are very few vegan-friendly foods that are
a complete protein unto themselves, which
is why quinoa is so special. Its nutty flavour
also plays well in lots of dishes, just be sure
to give it a rinse first, as its natural coating
can be bitter.

## BUCKWHEAT

Buckwheat, which is gluten-free, is another
pseudo-grain, and is actually more closely
related to rhubarb than wheat, despite its
misleading name. Buckwheat flour is well
known for being used in traditional French
crêpes, but the groats (or whole-grain

version) are perfect for porridge. You can also find it in cracked or ground form, which cooks even faster. Buckwheat is loaded with magnesium, copper and manganese.

## MILLET

Another mineral-dense gluten-free grain, millet is a great substitute for couscous or polenta/cornmeal, with its light sweetness, similar to ground corn.

## AMARANTH

Amaranth, which is gluten-free, is a protein super star, and is a good source of important B vitamins, including folate. This pseudo-grain is like a smaller version of quinoa or millet and is best served immediately once cooked, as it gets very gelatinous the longer it stands.

## POLENTA/CORNMEAL

Polenta/cornmeal, which is gluten-free, is made of dried ground corn and contains vitamins A and C. Its light sweetness and creamy texture make it a great foil for lots of different toppings. Though traditionally served in a savoury manner, it's also great with fruit, nuts, honey and maple syrup.

## FARRO

Farro, which contains gluten, is an ancient form of wheat and can also be referred to as emmer or einkorn. It's a great source

of protein, niacin (B3), magnesium and zinc. Its hearty shape and nutty flavour make it a great grain for adding to salads and soups, and it brings a great texture to porridges.

## RICE

I use both brown rice and black rice in this book, both of which are gluten-free. They are great sources of protein, fibre and minerals, with black rice slightly edging out brown rice in the antioxidant department.

## BARLEY

Barley, which contains gluten, is packed with selenium and B vitamins, so this grain can help balance hormones, along with a whole slew of other preventative health benefits. This whole grain is a great addition to both soups and porridges, just be aware of its longer cook time.

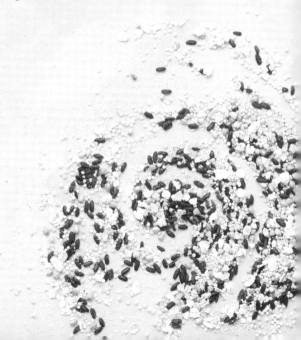

# GRAIN ALTERNATIVES

SOMETIMES WE CAN HAVE TOO MUCH OF A GOOD THING – EVEN
GRAINS. I FIND THAT WHEN I'M EATING GRAINS WITH EVERY MEAL FOR
AN EXTENDED PERIOD OF TIME, MY BODY CRAVES A BREAK. THESE
FOODS OFFER A SIMILAR COSY AND PORRIDGE-LIKE TEXTURE, ARE EASY
ON THE DIGESTIVE SYSTEM AND ARE NATURALLY GLUTEN-FREE.

## SWEET POTATO

Packed with vitamins A, C, and a bunch of
Bs, mashed sweet potatoes can go savoury
or sweet, and make a lovely grain-free
morning carbohydrate boost, along with all
the benefits of antioxidant-rich brightly
coloured veg.

## BUTTERNUT SQUASH

Similar to sweet potato in benefits, butternut
squash has a slightly less starchy quality.
When mashed with herb butter (like in the
Butternut Purée Porridge on page 131), it's
perfect for any meal.

## FLAX SEEDS/LINSEEDS

Flax seeds/linseeds are a great plant-based
source of omega-3 fatty acids, which help
with everything from skin issues to digestion.
Make sure to buy ground flax seeds/linseeds
(or grind them yourself), so you can actually
absorb their benefits. Store them in the
fridge in a dark container if possible, to keep
them fresh. They make a great addition
to any porridge and can absorb excess
moisture if you've added too much liquid.

## LENTILS

Lentils are plant-based protein powerhouses.
Red lentils can lend a particularly creamy,
porridge-like texture to dishes.

## CHIA SEEDS

Omega-3s, antioxidants and fibre are just
some of the major nutrients that chia seeds
bring to the table. They take on a slightly
weird, gelatinous texture when they absorb
liquid, but if you're into that sort of thing
(and I must admit, it really grows on you!),
you'll love these little seeds.

## MAKE THEM MORE DELICIOUS

To turn these grain alternatives into a
comforting porridge, make sure you add
extra richness – use a good quality fat like
coconut cream, butter or nut butters. Spices
or herbs also help to give these ingredients
a more robust sweet or savoury flavour.

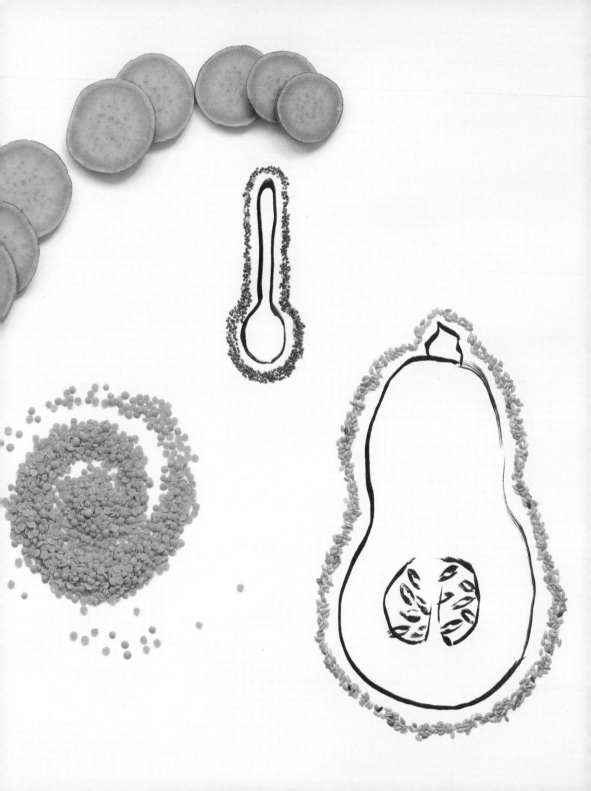

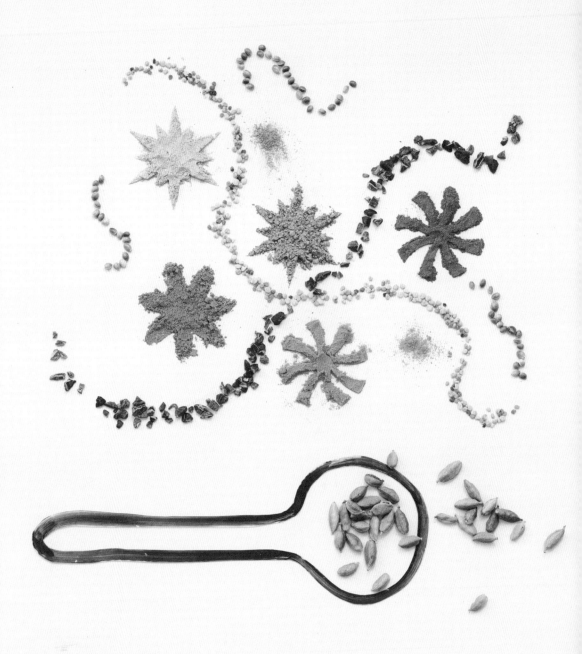

# ADAPTOGENS, SUPERFOODS AND SUPER SPICES

THESE ARE THE ADD-ONS THAT CAN BRING SOME BIG NUTRITIONAL BENEFITS.
AS SOME OF THESE CAN BE PRICEY, MOST AREN'T 100% NECESSARY IN THE RECIPES
(WITH THE EXCEPTION OF SPICES), BUT I WILL NOTE WHERE YOU CAN USE THEM.

## MACA

Great for hormone-balancing and natural energy.

## MATCHA

This antioxidant-packed powder is supercharged green tea – it's essentially the tea leaves ground up, so you're getting the maximum benefits of consuming the whole leaf. It's great for a calm caffeine buzz that doesn't make you shaky.

## ASHWAGANDHA

This anti-inflammatory can be helpful for reducing stress and improving mood.

## HEMP SEEDS

These super seeds are a great plant-based source of omega-3 fatty acids and protein. They're mild in flavour and easy to sprinkle on almost anything.

## CACAO

Cacao comes in powder and nibs, and is another natural energy-booster. It also brings a good dose of antioxidants, as well as magnesium, which can help relax muscles and promote healthy digestion.

## BEE POLLEN

With protein, B vitamins and antioxidants, these little granules can pack a punch. However, if you have an allergy to pollen, please don't reach for this one.

## TURMERIC

Known for its anti-inflammatory properties, this spice can help reduce pain and boost brain power. It's more easily absorbed when consumed with a pinch of black pepper.

## CINNAMON

Antioxidant, anti-inflammatory and heart-protective, this spice also adds natural sweetness sans sugar, keeps your blood sugar in check.

## CARDAMOM

In addition to its anti-inflammatory qualities, it also helps soothe stomach issues, and can help freshen your breath. It's also naturally sweet, so a great addition to porridges.

# PROTEIN ADD-INS

PROTEIN HELPS US FEEL FULLER FOR LONGER AND PROVIDES US WITH ENERGY TO POWER THROUGH OUR DAYS. THE GOOD NEWS IS GRAINS ALREADY CONTAIN PROTEIN, BUT TO GIVE YOUR MORNING AN EXTRA BOOST, TRY ADDING ONE OF THESE TO YOUR BOWL.

## SUNFLOWER SEED BUTTER

A great option for anyone with nut allergies, or if you're just looking to mix it up. You can use it as a substitute for almond or peanut butter in several recipes. I like to add a little vanilla and cinnamon to mine (see recipe on page 25) to add some sweet flavours.

## ALMOND BUTTER

Filled with vitamin E and vital minerals such as calcium and magnesium, almond butter is great for skin and bone health. Its mild flavour makes it a happy addition to many different bowls.

## HAZELNUT BUTTER

Another nut that is teeming with vitamins and minerals, the hazelnut can help improve heart and brain health. Use this nutty spread for nutella-esque flavours. See recipe on page 26.

## PEANUT BUTTER

Peanut butter is a classic lunchbox staple that brings a distinct nostalgia to anything it touches. Its flavour is strong, but that is often a good thing. Try it in the Chocolate Peanut Butter Chia Pots (page 104).

## ALMOND FLOUR

This is a great add-in to boost the protein in your porridge. You can stir in a couple of tablespoons into most warm porridges (especially sweet ones) for a mellow, nutty flavour and an extra fibre boost.

## EGGS

Eggs are an excellent source of protein, selenium, B vitamins and so much more, so if you're not a vegan, add these guys to your savoury porridges. They're versatile too – fry, boil, poach or scramble to suit your mood.

# MILK ALTERNATIVES

FOR THE DAIRY-ADVERSE OR THOSE LOOKING TO CUT BACK ON ANIMAL PRODUCTS, MILK ALTERNATIVES ARE A GREAT PLACE TO START ESPECIALLY IN PORRIDGE. THESE PLANT-BASED MILKS LEND CREAMINESS AND FLAVOUR WITHOUT THE LACTOSE.

## ALMOND MILK

This is one of the most neutral plant-based milks I've come across, but the type you buy matters. I try to get the kind that has the fewest ingredients, avoiding sweeteners and thickeners (like carrageenan), if possible. Carrageenan is extracted from seaweed, and is often used as a thickener. It's been linked to digestive issues and inflammation, so if you're consuming almond milk regularly, it's best to avoid it. You can also make your own almond milk (page 22) that contains more fibre and protein than store-bought versions, without any soaking or straining.

## COCONUT MILK

Coconut milk is the thickest plant-based milk and it is easily available. I usually just buy cans of it and mix it with water to thin out the consistency and make it last longer. I combine a 400-g/14-oz. can of coconut milk with a can's worth of filtered water, and use a stick blender to get rid of any clumps. Again, try to find one that doesn't have gums or thickeners – you don't need 'em!

## HEMP MILK

You can also easily make your own hemp milk, without any straining, for a big boost of omega-3 fatty acids.

## CASHEW MILK

This nut-based milk can either be on the creamier, thick side or the thinner side depending on how much water you use to blend it with. I don't strain mine, so I make sure to blend it at the maximum speed for at least a few minutes. Start with a thicker version and add more water to get the consistency you want.

# CREATIVE TOPPINGS

PORRIDGE IS A GREAT BLANK CANVAS FOR ALL TYPES OF TOPPINGS. HERE ARE SOME OF MY FAVOURITE WAYS TO INCORPORATE THEM FOR BEAUTIFUL BOWLS THAT TASTE AS GOOD AS THEY LOOK.

## GET CREATIVE

Whether you're trying to add some extra flavour, sweetness, or colour, don't feel boxed in! Take stock of what you have – whether it's fresh or frozen fruit, nuts and seeds, granola, edible flower petals, dairy or nut cheese – and give it a try! Sometimes I'll fall back on classic flavour pairings, but other times it's great to break the mould and try something new.

## CHANGE YOUR CONTAINER

Bowls of all shapes and sizes are lovely, but give a wide-mouthed glass jar or shallow cup a try. Cold porridges are great for popping in glass jars to grab and go.

## LAYER IT

Layering goes well with porridges served in glass jars or cups, and makes your porridge both visually and texturally interesting, with topping flavours throughout. Try adding a layer of nut butter, granola or berries (or all three!) halfway through your porridge. You could even layer two different types of porridge for different flavours and colours.

The smoothie-overnight oats hybrids, (pages 96, 103 and 108) would be great for this.

## THINK TEXTURE

Porridge texture can sometimes be a little one-note. Its essence is creamy and mushy, so toppings serve as a great contrast to that. Think about what will add a little pop, crunch or chewiness to the bowl. Nuts and seeds are, of course, great for this, but look to raspberries and blackberries for a fibre-filled pop, and naturally sweet toasted coconut and thinly shaved raw vegetables for a fresh crunchiness. Add chewiness with dried fruits and roasted vegetables.

## BRING OUT YOUR ARTISTIC SIDE

Lastly, think about the design when making up a bowl of porridge. This might sound a little ambitious, but we eat with our eyes first, so it's a great way to exercise your creativity and find out what you respond to. Try arranging toppings in concentric circles or in a layered half-moon on one side of the bowl, or add a Jackson Pollock-like lashing of almond butter to your masterpiece.

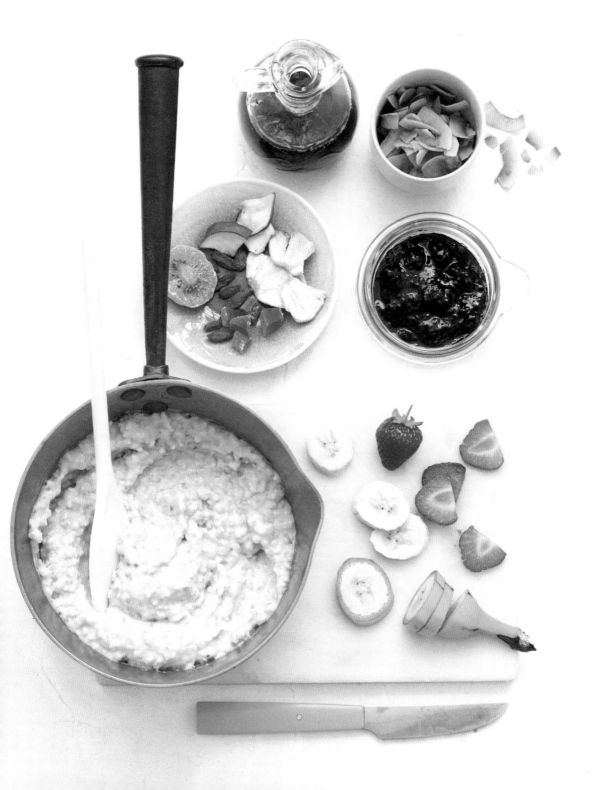

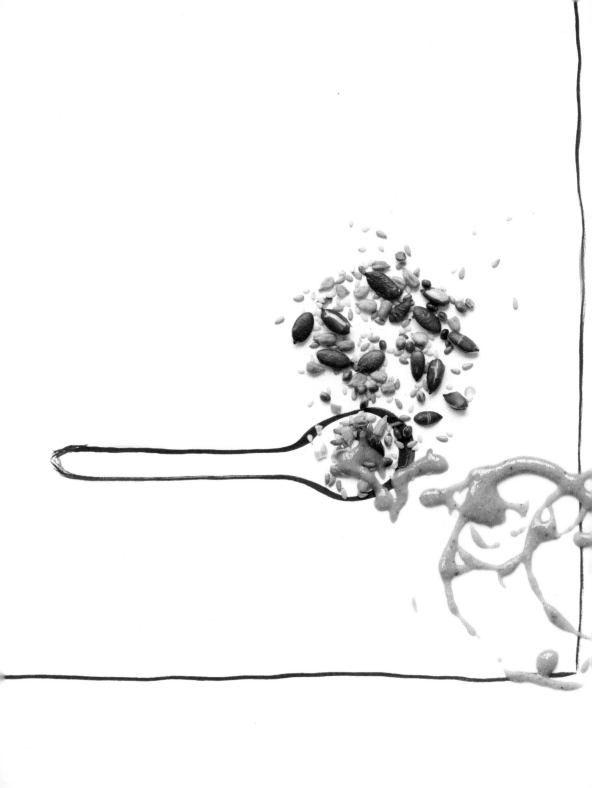

# BASIC
# RECIPES
# AND
# TOPPINGS

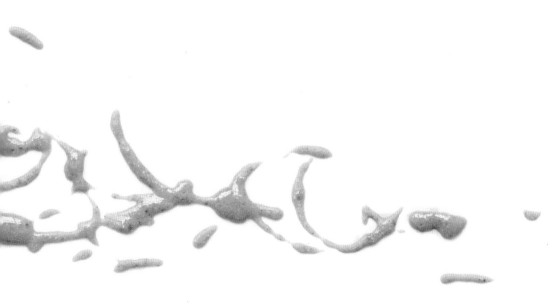

# NUT MILKS

MAKING YOUR OWN NUT MILK SOUNDS HARD, BUT HERE ARE THREE RECIPES THAT IGNORE THE RULES ABOUT STRAINING AND EXCESSIVE SOAKING IN FAVOUR OF SIMPLICITY.

**LAZY ALMOND MILK**

**3 tablespoons almond butter**

**500 ml/2 cups water**

**pinch of sea salt**

**HEMP MILK**

**55 g/½ cup hemp seeds**

**500 ml/2 cups filtered water**

**pinch of sea salt**

**CASHEW MILK**

**120 g/1 cup raw cashews, soaked in 500 ml/2 cups water for at least 2 hours or overnight, then drained**

**3 dates, stoned/pitted and soaked**

**pinch of sea salt**

**500–750 ml/2–3 cups water (separate from the soaking water)**

MAKES ABOUT 500 ML/2 CUPS

LAZY ALMOND MILK

In a blender, process all the ingredients on high for 1–3 minutes until the almond butter is well combined with the water. Store in the refrigerator in an airtight jar for up to 4–5 days and shake before using.

HEMP MILK

Put everything in a blender and purée until smooth. This can take a couple of minutes, depending on your blender. Store in an airtight jar in the refrigerator for up to 7 days and shake before using.

CASHEW MILK

Start by blending the soaked and drained cashews with the dates and salt into a fine paste, then gradually add 500 ml/2 cups water and blend until smooth. You can add more water for a thinner consistency. Store in the refrigerator in an airtight jar for up to 5 days and shake before using.

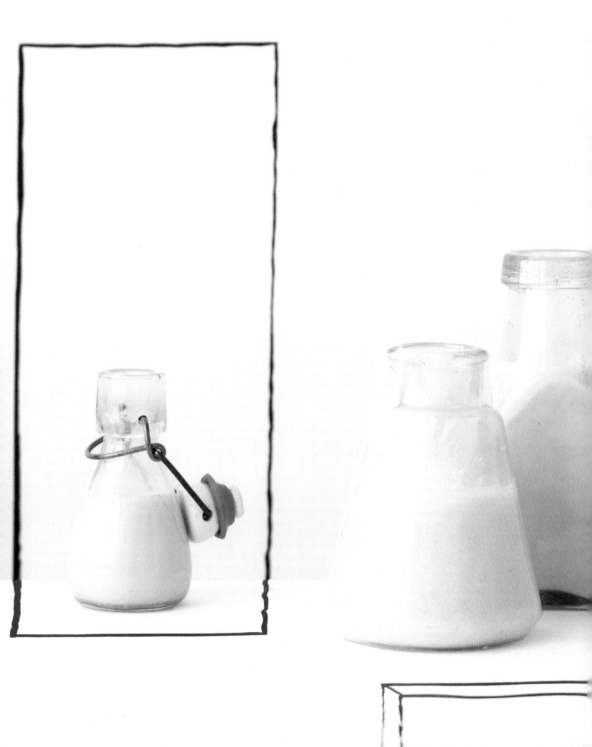

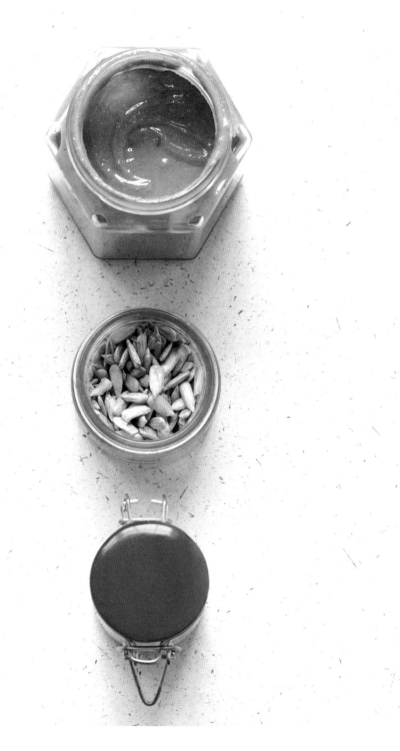

# SUNFLOWER SEED BUTTER

IF YOU HAVE A NUT ALLERGY OR JUST WANT TO MIX THINGS UP
WITH SOME SEEDS, GIVE THIS SUNFLOWER SEED BUTTER A TRY. I ADD
GROUND CINNAMON AND VANILLA EXTRACT HERE TO GIVE IT A RICH AND
NATURALLY SWEET FLAVOUR.

**280 g/2 cups raw shelled sunflower
seeds**

**½ teaspoon pure vanilla extract**

**½ teaspoon ground cinnamon
(optional)**

**pinch of sea salt**

**1 tablespoon neutral-tasting oil,
such as grape seed oil or sunflower/
safflower oil**

MAKES ABOUT 300 G/1¼ CUPS

Preheat the oven to 180°C (350°F) Gas 4.

Place the seeds on a baking sheet in a single layer
and bake in the preheated oven for 5–8 minutes until
lightly toasted. Watch them closely as these can burn
easily, especially if you have a hot oven.

Allow the seeds to cool completely before
transferring to a food processor or high-speed
blender. Add the vanilla, cinnamon and salt and
blend. Once you have a rough paste (after 6–7
minutes of blending), slowly add the neutral oil while
the blades are going.

Blend for 8–12 minutes in total, possibly more,
depending on your machine. Have patience, you will
get a seed butter eventually. You'll have to scrape
down the sides a few times, to make sure everything
is getting incorporated.

Store in the refrigerator in an airtight jar for up to
a month.

# NUT BUTTERS

FANCY NUT BUTTERS CAN GET EXPENSIVE. WITH A BLENDER OR FOOD PROCESSOR AND SOME PATIENCE, YOU CAN MAKE YOUR OWN.

**HAZELNUT BUTTER**

**130 g/1 cup hazelnuts, skins removed**

**1 tablespoon neutral-tasting oil, such as grape seed oil or sunflower/ safflower oil**

**1 teaspoon pure vanilla extract**

**pinch of sea salt**

**2 tablespoons unsweetened cocoa or cacao powder (optional)**

MAKES ABOUT 150 G/¾ CUP

**CASHEW BUTTER**

**240 g/2 cups raw cashews**

**pinch of sea salt**

**1 tablespoon neutral-tasting oil, such as grape seed oil or sunflower/ safflower oil**

MAKES ABOUT 250 G/1¼ CUPS

## HAZELNUT BUTTER

Process the hazelnuts in a food processor or high-speed blender for 8–12 minutes, depending on your machine. First you'll get a fine powder, but continue blending until you get a denser, softened nut butter.

Add the oil, vanilla, salt and cocoa or cacao powder (if using) and process to combine for 2–4 minutes until smooth. Depending on your food processor or blender, the consistency may vary. Store in the refrigerator in an airtight jar for up to a month.

## CASHEW BUTTER

Preheat the oven to 180°C (350°F) Gas 4.

Place the cashews on a baking sheet in a single layer and bake in the preheated oven for 6–9 minutes until lightly toasted. Keep an eye on them to make sure they don't burn.

Allow the cashews to cool completely before transferring to a food processor or high-speed blender. Add the salt and blend. Once you have a rough paste (after 6–7 minutes of blending), slowly add the neutral oil while the blades are going. Blend for 8–12 minutes in total, possibly more, depending on your machine. Have patience, you will get a nut butter eventually. You'll have to scrape down the sides a few times, to make sure everything is getting incorporated. Store in the refrigerator in an airtight jar for up to a month.

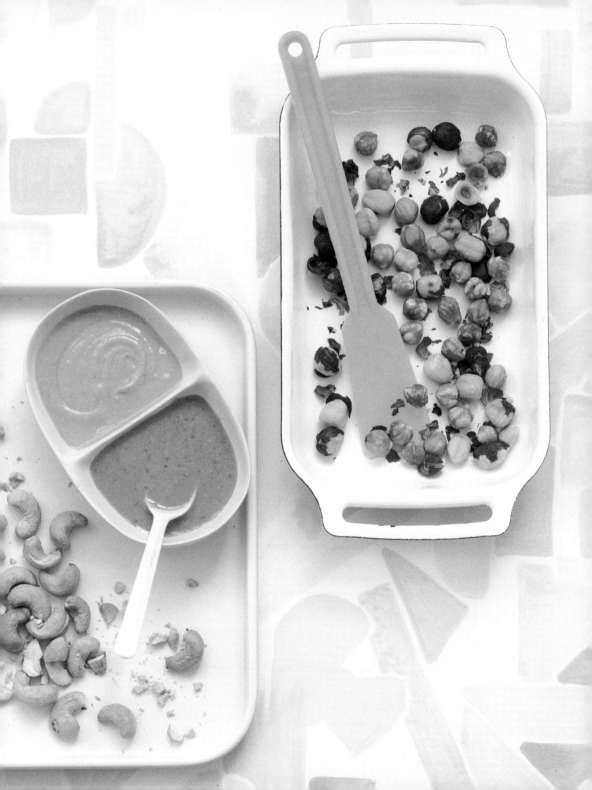

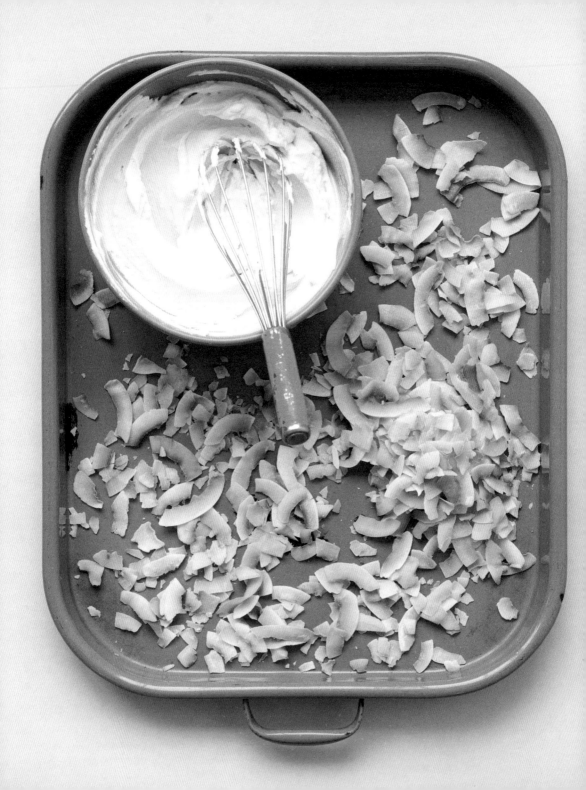

# COCONUT WHIPPED CREAM

THE DAIRY-FREE ANSWER TO WHIPPED CREAM, A SPOONFUL OF THIS WILL MAKE A PORRIDGE FEEL EXTRA SPECIAL.

**400-g/14-oz. can full-fat coconut milk, cooled in the refrigerator overnight**

**1 teaspoon pure maple syrup**

**¼ teaspoon pure vanilla extract or paste**

## MAKES ABOUT 125 ML/½ CUP

Put a mixing bowl in the freezer about 5 minutes before you start.

Scoop out the hardened coconut cream from the top of the can, reserving the coconut water for something else (like a smoothie), and place the cream in the chilled mixing bowl.

Whip, using an electric whisk or beaters, until light and airy with little to no clumps, about 1–2 minutes. Add the maple syrup and vanilla, and whisk again for about 1 minute more to distribute evenly. Use immediately or store in an airtight jar in the refrigerator for up to 3 days.

# TOASTED COCONUT

WITH A SATISFYING CRUNCH AND DEEP COCONUT FLAVOUR, TAKING A LITTLE EXTRA TIME TO TOAST YOUR COCONUT FLAKES IS TOTALLY WORTH IT.

**45 g/1 cup large unsweetened dried coconut flakes**

*baking sheet lined with baking parchment*

## MAKES 45 G/1 CUP

Preheat the oven to 180°C (350°F) Gas 4.

Spread the coconut flakes out on the lined baking sheet. Bake for 3–5 minutes until golden. Watch the coconut flakes closely, as these can burn very quickly.

Leave to cool. Store in an airtight jar or container at room temperature for up to 2 weeks.

# TOASTED SEEDS AND NUTS

TOASTING NUTS AND SEEDS UPS THEIR CRUNCH FACTOR, MAKES THEM EASIER TO DIGEST AND ENHANCES THEIR NATURAL FLAVOURS — WHAT'S NOT TO LOVE?

**130 g/1 cup raw nuts or seeds**

MAKES 130 G/1 CUP

Preheat the oven to 180°C (350°F) Gas 4.

Spread the nuts or seeds out on a baking sheet. For nuts, bake in the preheated oven for 6–8 minutes. For seeds, bake for 3–5 minutes. Leave to cool.

Store in an airtight jar in the refrigerator for up to three months.

**Note:** Pay attention – all ovens are different and seeds and nuts can go from golden to burned pretty quickly, so keep a close eye on them.

# DUKKAH

DUKKAH IS AN EGYPTIAN CONDIMENT, WHICH CAN BE USED ON SCRAMBLED EGGS, PORRIDGE OR SALADS.

**30 g/¼ cup shelled pistachios, roughly chopped**

**30 g/¼ cup almonds, roughly chopped**

**1 tablespoon cumin seeds**

**1 tablespoon coriander seeds**

**1 tablespoon sesame seeds**

**1 teaspoon sea salt**

**1 teaspoon cracked black pepper**

**½ teaspoon dried chilli flakes/hot red pepper flakes**

MAKES ABOUT 100 G/½–¾ CUP

Heat a large frying pan/skillet over a medium heat. Add the nuts, and dry toast for 5 minutes, tossing occasionally, until they're starting to turn golden and fragrant. Transfer to a plate. In the same pan, toast the cumin, coriander and sesame seeds for 2–4 minutes over a medium-low heat, until fragrant.

Combine the nuts, seeds, salt, pepper and dried chilli flakes/hot red pepper flakes in a small food processor or clean coffee grinder, until finely chopped into small bits and pieces that still lend a bit of crunch. Store in an airtight glass container in the refrigerator for 3 months.

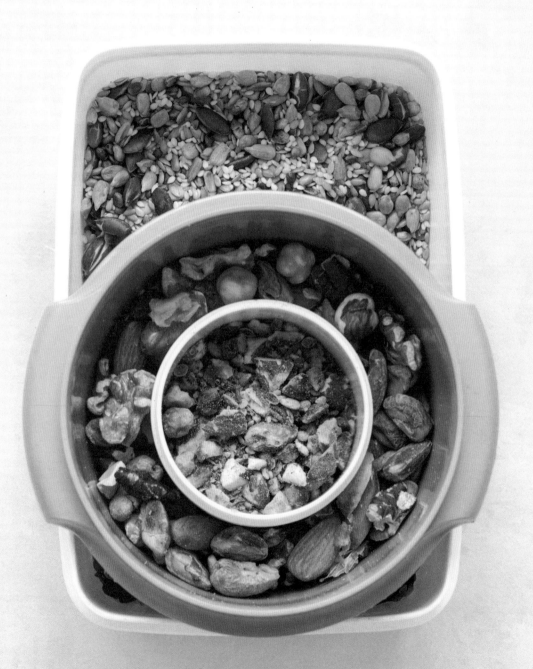

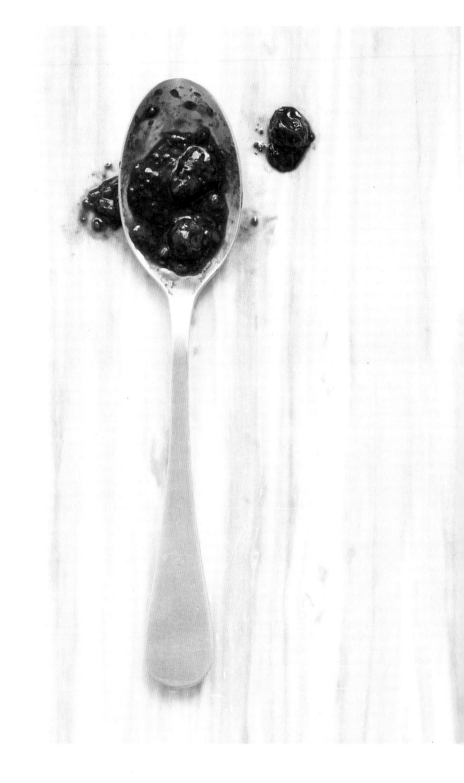

# BERRY COMPOTE

I SUGGEST FROZEN BERRIES FOR THIS RECIPE FOR A COUPLE OF REASONS: FIRSTLY, IF BERRIES ARE IN SEASON, I PREFER TO HAVE THEM FRESH AND RARELY COOK THEM. SECONDLY, WHEN BERRIES AREN'T IN SEASON, FROZEN OPTIONS ARE CHEAPER AND OFTEN TASTE BETTER.

**375 g/2 cups frozen berries (blueberries and raspberries work especially well for this; you can also use a mix if you prefer)**

**125 ml/½ cup water, plus more as needed**

**2 teaspoons chia seeds**

**1 tablespoon sweetener (honey, maple syrup, muscovado or demerara/ turbinado sugar)**

**1 tablespoon freshly squeezed lemon juice**

## MAKES ABOUT 400 ML/ 1¾ CUPS

Combine everything together in a medium saucepan and bring to a simmer over a medium-low heat. Simmer for 10 minutes, stirring frequently, until jammy and sweet. If the pan gets dry at any point, add a small splash of water.

Leave to cool. Store in an airtight container in the refrigerator for up to 5 days.

# ROASTED STONE FRUIT

A BASIC METHOD FOR ROASTED FRUIT, YOU CAN EASILY DOUBLE
OR TRIPLE THIS, JUST MAKE SURE EACH PIECE HAS SPACE ON THE BAKING
SHEET. THIS IS GREAT AS A TOPPER FOR PORRIDGE, OF COURSE, BUT
ALSO AS A DESSERT WITH ICE CREAM OR WHIPPED CREAM. THERE
IS A SIMILAR VERSION IN THE MILLET PORRIDGE WITH THYME-ROASTED
PLUMS ON PAGE 76.

**2 peaches or other stone fruit (such
as plums or apricots), cut in half and
stoned/pitted**

*baking sheet lined with baking
parchment*

SERVES 2

Preheat the oven to 190°C (375°F) Gas 5.

Place the peaches or other stone fruit, skin-side down
(cut-side up), on the lined baking sheet.

Roast in the preheated oven for 10–15 minutes, until
fragrant and juicy.

Leave to cool. Store in an airtight container in the
refrigerator for up to 5 days.

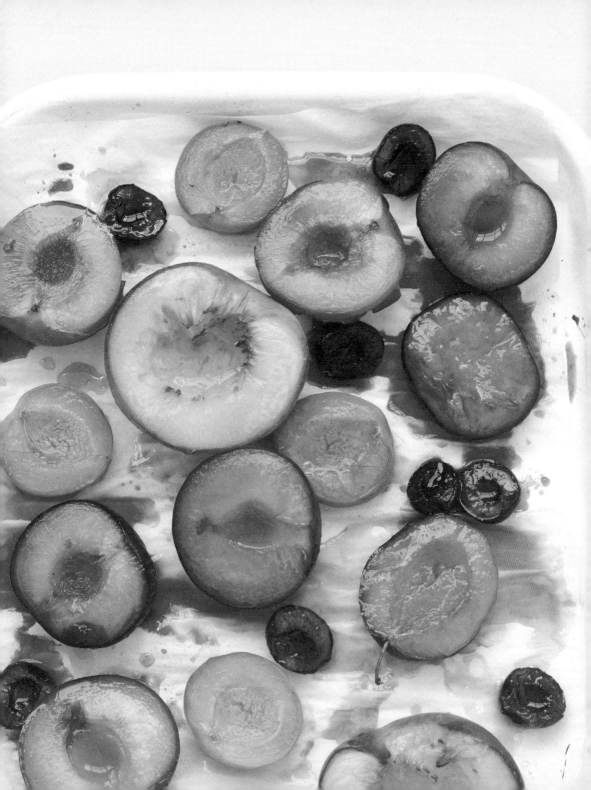

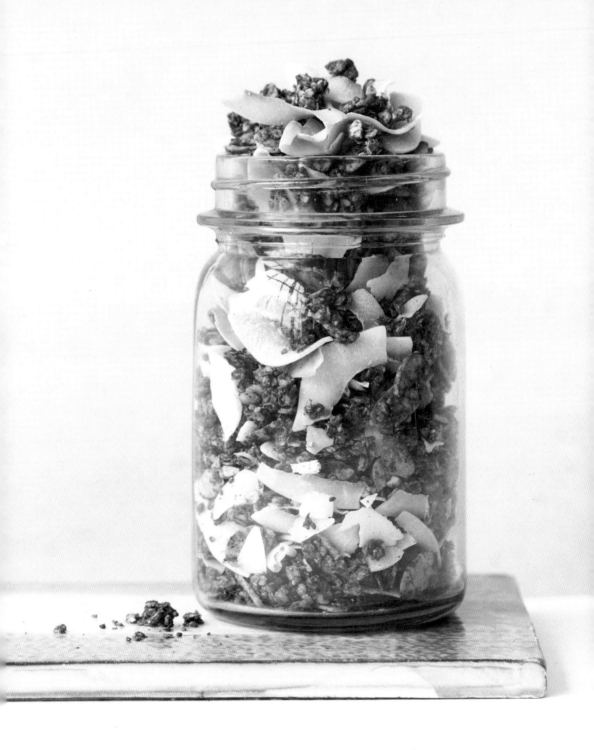

# CHOCOLATE AND COCONUT GRANOLA

IF YOU LOVE YOUR BREAKFAST ON THE SWEET AND CRUNCHY SIDE, MAKING YOUR OWN GRANOLA IS ONE OF THE EASIEST AND MOST SATISFYING THINGS YOU SHOULD MASTER. THIS VERSION MADE WITH CACAO TASTES LIKE GROWN-UP COCO POPS.

**190 g/2 cups rolled/old-fashioned oats**

**80 g/1 cup flaked/sliced almonds (substitute sunflower or pumpkin seeds for a nut-free version)**

**4 tablespoons cacao powder**

**2 tablespoons chia seeds**

**½ teaspoon sea salt**

**1 tablespoon maca powder (optional)**

**60 ml/¼ cup melted coconut oil**

**60 ml/¼ cup pure maple syrup**

**45 g/1 cup coconut flakes**

***baking sheet lined with baking parchment***

## MAKES ABOUT 500 G/3½ CUPS

Preheat the oven to 160°C (325°F) Gas 3.

In a large mixing bowl, combine the oats, almonds, cacao powder, chia seeds, salt and maca (if using). Mix together to distribute the cacao evenly.

In a pourable glass measuring jug/cup, combine the oil and maple syrup, and whisk together with a fork. Pour the wet ingredients into the dry and mix together until the oats are evenly coated.

Spread out in an even layer on the prepared baking sheet and bake in the oven for 20 minutes. Take out the sheet, rotate it 180 degrees, sprinkle the coconut flakes on top and bake for another 15–20 minutes.

Note: If you smell burning at any point, take out the baking sheet to cool a little, stir the mixture and turn the oven down slightly. Return to the oven for the remainder of the cooking time or a little less.

Remove from the oven and leave to cool completely on the baking sheet – this is when it will really crisp up and get its crunch. Once cooled, break into pieces and store in an airtight jar at room temperature for up to 2 weeks, or in the refrigerator for up to 1 month.

# CARDAMOM TAHINI GRANOLA

TAHINI IS MADE FROM GROUND SESAME SEEDS AND LENDS A NUTTY AND SLIGHTLY BITTER TASTE TO THIS GRANOLA THAT PAIRS PERFECTLY WITH FRAGRANT AND SWEET CARDAMOM.

**240 g/2½ cups rolled/old-fashioned oats**

**65 g/½ cup walnut pieces or roughly chopped walnuts**

**65 g/½ cup shelled pistachios (or substitute another nut or seed of your choice)**

**2 tablespoons chia seeds**

**1 teaspoon ground cinnamon**

**½–1 teaspoon ground cardamom, to taste**

**¼ teaspoon sea salt**

**60 ml/¼ cup melted coconut oil**

**60 g/¼ cup tahini**

**60 ml/¼ cup pure maple syrup or honey**

*baking sheet lined with baking parchment*

MAKES ABOUT 500 G/3½ CUPS

Preheat the oven to 160°C (325°F) Gas 3.

In a large mixing bowl, combine the oats, walnuts, pistachios, chia seeds, cinnamon, cardamom and salt. Mix together to distribute the spices evenly.

In a pourable glass measuring jug/cup, combine the melted coconut oil, tahini and maple syrup, and mix together with a fork. Pour the wet ingredients into the dry and mix together with a silicone spatula until the oats are evenly coated in the coconut tahini mixture.

Spread the oat mixture out in an even layer on the prepared baking sheet and bake in the oven for 20 minutes. Take out the baking sheet, rotate it 180 degrees, and bake for another 15–20 minutes until golden but not too brown.

Remove from the oven and leave to cool completely on the baking sheet – this is when it will really crisp up and get its crunch. Once cooled, break into pieces and store in an airtight jar at room temperature for up to 2 weeks, or in the refrigerator for up to 1 month.

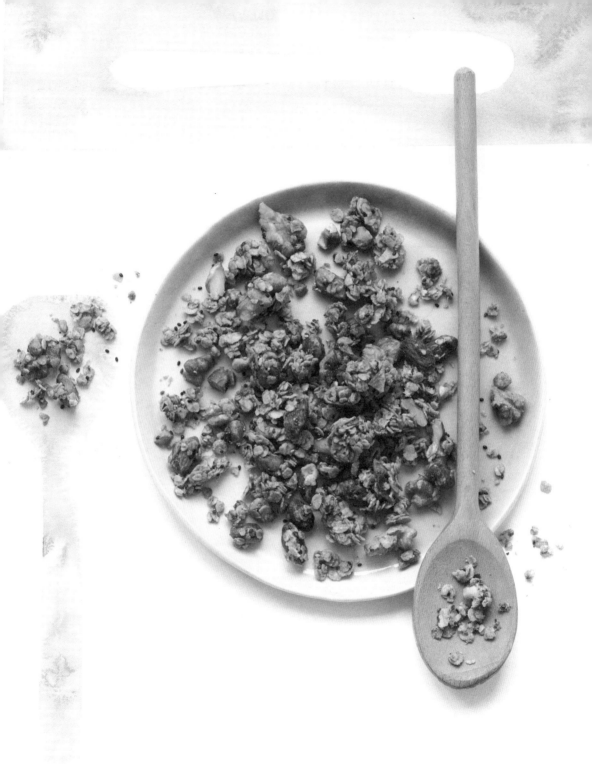

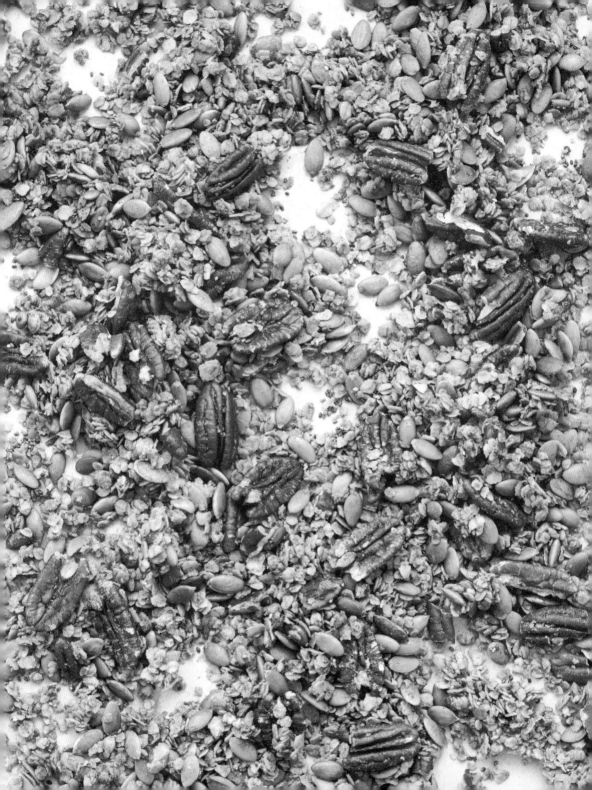

# MAPLE PECAN GRANOLA

MAPLE PECAN GRANOLA IS THE MOST CLASSIC OF THESE GRANOLA
RECIPES AND ONE OF MY FAVOURITES FOR TOPPING EVERYTHING FROM
WARM AND COLD PORRIDGES TO DESSERTS MADE WITH WARM BAKED
FRUIT. GRANOLA MAKES A GREAT HOSTESS GIFT, TOO.

**285 g/3 cups rolled/old-fashioned oats**

**100 g/1 cup pecan pieces**

**140 g/1 cup pumpkin seeds/pepitas**

**2 tablespoons chia seeds**

**2 teaspoons ground cinnamon**

**½ teaspoon sea salt**

**125 ml/½ cup avocado or olive oil**

**125 ml/½ cup pure maple syrup**

**1 teaspoon pure vanilla extract**

*baking sheet lined with baking
parchment*

## MAKES ABOUT 650 G/5 CUPS

Preheat the oven to 160°C (325°F) Gas 3.

In a large mixing bowl, combine the oats, pecans,
pumpkin seeds/pepitas, chia seeds, cinnamon and
salt. Mix together to distribute the ingredients evenly.

In a pourable glass measuring jug/cup, combine the
oil, maple syrup and vanilla and mix together with
a fork. Pour the wet ingredients into the dry and mix
together until the oats are evenly coated.

Spread in an even layer on the prepared baking sheet
and bake in the oven for 20 minutes. Take out the
baking sheet, rotate it 180 degrees, and bake for
another 15–20 minutes until golden but not too brown.

Remove from the oven and leave to cool completely
on the baking sheet – this is when it will really crisp
up and get its crunch. Once cooled, break into pieces
and store in an airtight jar at room temperature for
up to 2 weeks, or in the refrigerator for up to 1 month.

# RED PESTO

THIS UMAMI-RICH SUN-DRIED TOMATO PESTO IS PACKED WITH MEDITERRANEAN FLAVOUR. IT ADDS AN ALMOST PIZZA-TASTING VIBE TO SAVOURY DISHES — IN THE BEST POSSIBLE WAY.

**225 g/8 oz. oil-packed sun-dried tomatoes**

**125 ml/½ cup olive oil (this can include oil from the jar of tomatoes)**

**1 garlic clove, peeled**

**30 g/¼ cup cashews or pine nuts, toasted**

**1 tablespoon freshly squeezed lemon juice**

**pinch of dried chilli flakes/hot red pepper flakes**

**sea salt, to taste**

## MAKES ABOUT 300 G/1 CUP

Place the sun-dried tomatoes, half the olive oil, the garlic, cashews or pine nuts, lemon juice, dried chilli flakes/hot red pepper flakes and a generous pinch of salt in a food processor.

Blitz until a rough paste forms and then, with the processor running, add the remaining olive oil until you get a smooth-ish purée.

Store in an airtight jar for 3–4 days in the refrigerator or in the freezer for up to 3 months.

# GREEN PESTO

A SIMPLE BASIL PESTO IS AN EASY WAY TO PERK UP A SAVOURY PORRIDGE OR ANY TYPE OF GRAIN BOWL. IF YOU CAN GET YOUR HANDS ON A BUNCH OF FRESH BASIL, YOU'RE HALFWAY THERE.

**40 g/2 packed cups basil leaves**

**60 g/½ cup pine nuts or cashews (or a mix)**

**1 garlic clove, peeled**

**20 g/¼ cup grated Parmesan (substitute 2 tablespoons nutritional yeast for a vegan version)**

**1 teaspoon freshly squeezed lemon juice**

**60–125 ml/¼–½ cup olive oil**

## MAKES ABOUT 200 G/1 CUP

In a food processor or blender, combine the basil, pine nuts or cashews, garlic, Parmesan and lemon juice, and pulse until everything is finely chopped, scraping down the sides a couple of times with a silicone spatula.

With the motor running on low, slowly pour in the olive oil, adding more oil for a thinner pesto if you prefer.

Store in an airtight jar for 3–4 days in the refrigerator or in the freezer for up to 3 months.

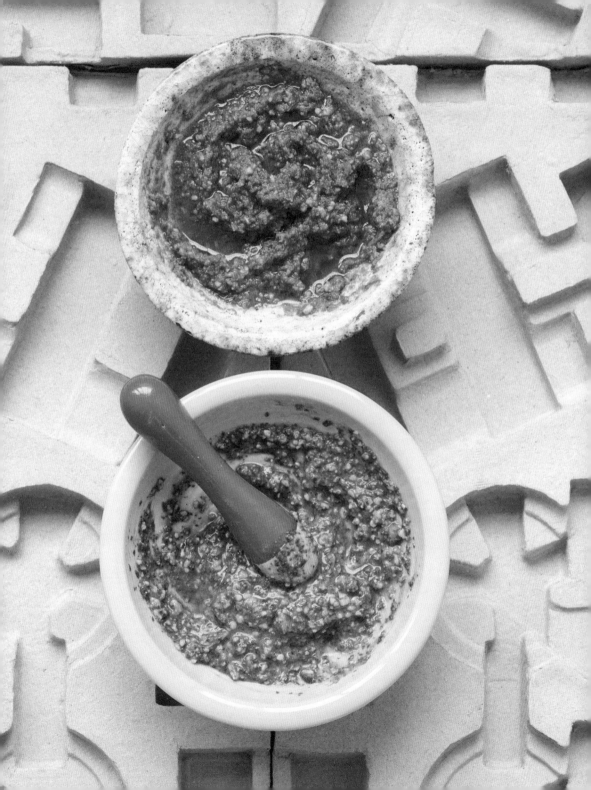

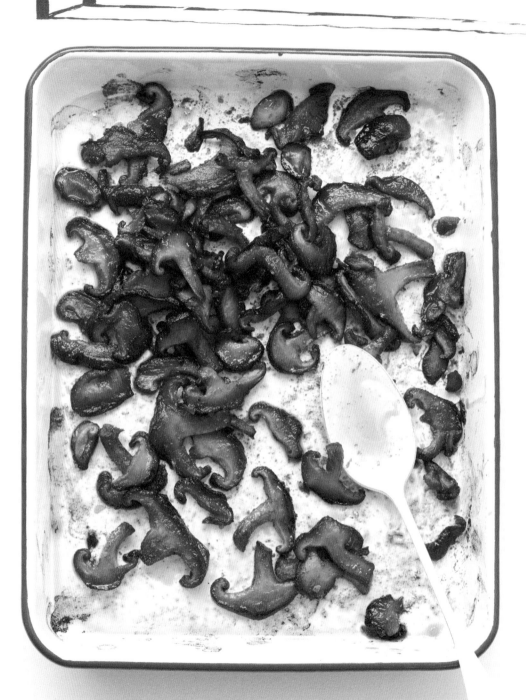

# SHIITAKE MUSHROOM 'BACON'

I'M NOT TRYING TO REPLACE BACON, BUT RATHER OFFER A SMOKY
PLANT-BASED ALTERNATIVE THAT'S DELICIOUS IN ITS OWN RIGHT. WITH
SMOKED PAPRIKA AND A HINT OF MAPLE, THIS ALMOST-MEATY
VEGETABLE GETS A BREAKFAST-WORTHY MAKEOVER.

**2 tablespoons avocado or other
neutral oil**

**2 teaspoons sweet smoked paprika**

**1 tablespoon tamari**

**1 teaspoon pure maple syrup**

**150 g/5 oz. fresh shiitake mushrooms,
sliced**

**sea salt or smoked sea salt, to taste**

MAKES ABOUT 150 G/1 CUP

Preheat the grill/broiler to high.

In a medium mixing bowl, whisk the oil, paprika,
tamari, maple syrup and a pinch or two of salt
together. Add the sliced mushrooms to the mixing
bowl and toss to coat them in the spiced oil.

Spread the mushrooms out on a baking sheet and
place under the grill/broiler for 4–5 minutes. Rotate
the sheet and cook for another 1–2 minutes until
crispy around the edges. Keep an eye on them,
as grills/broilers can be unpredictable.

Leave to cool on the baking sheet for 2–5 minutes,
taste for seasoning, and serve.

Store in an airtight container in the refrigerator
for up to 5 days. When ready to serve, re-crisp in a
cast-iron frying pan/skillet for 2 minutes on a medium-
high heat.

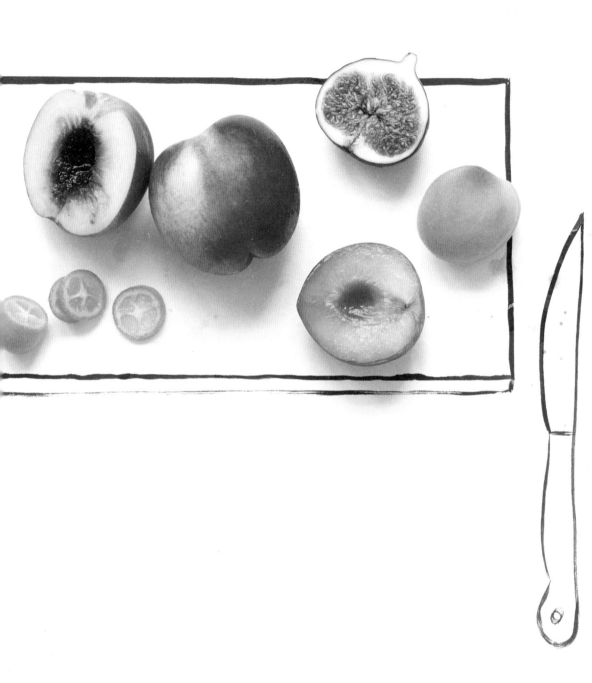

# SWEET
# AND
# WARMING

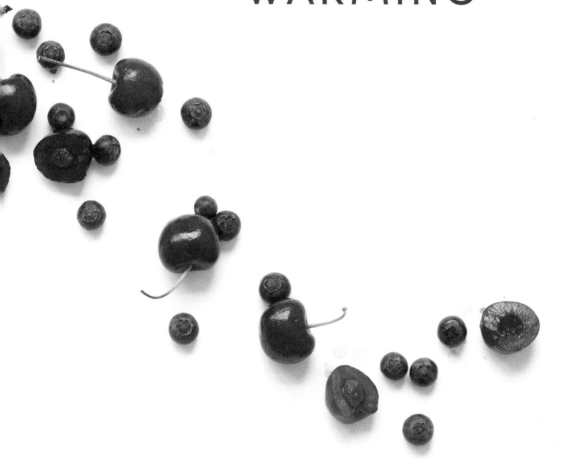

# CLASSIC MIXED OATMEAL PORRIDGE

THIS GENIUS YET SIMPLE COMBINATION OF COARSE OATMEAL/
STEEL-CUT OATS AND ROLLED/OLD-FASHIONED OATS CAME TO ME BY
WAY OF APRIL BLOOMFIELD IN HER BOOK 'A GIRL AND HER PIG'. IT GIVES
A CREAMY, YET TEXTURED CONSISTENCY THAT IS SUPER SATISFYING.

**70 g/½ cup coarse oatmeal/
steel-cut oats**

**50 g/½ cup rolled/old-fashioned oats**

**2 teaspoons apple cider vinegar**

**500 ml/2 cups water, plus more
for soaking**

**250 ml/1 cup milk of choice**

**¾ teaspoon salt**

**OPTIONAL TOPPINGS**

**Berry Compote (page 33)**

**Toasted Coconut (page 29)**

**sliced fresh fruit (such as banana,
strawberries or kiwi)**

**chopped dried fruit (such as
cranberries, pineapple or papaya)**

**add-ons for texture (such as pistachios,
chia seeds, bee pollen, freeze-dried
raspberries or blueberry powder)**

**brown sugar or pure maple syrup**

SERVES 2–3

The night before, combine both types of oatmeal/
oats with enough water to cover them by about
5 cm/2 inches and the apple cider vinegar. Leave
to sit at room temperature for at least 8 hours.

The next morning, drain the oats and rinse them.
Transfer to a medium saucepan and add the water,
milk and salt.

Bring to the boil, then reduce to a simmer. Cover
with the lid slightly ajar and cook for 10–15 minutes,
stirring occasionally. You want most of the liquid to be
absorbed but the mixture should be loose and not
gluey. If it's a little too thick for your liking, add more
water and milk, and stir in, cooking for a couple
of minutes more.

Serve with your desired toppings.

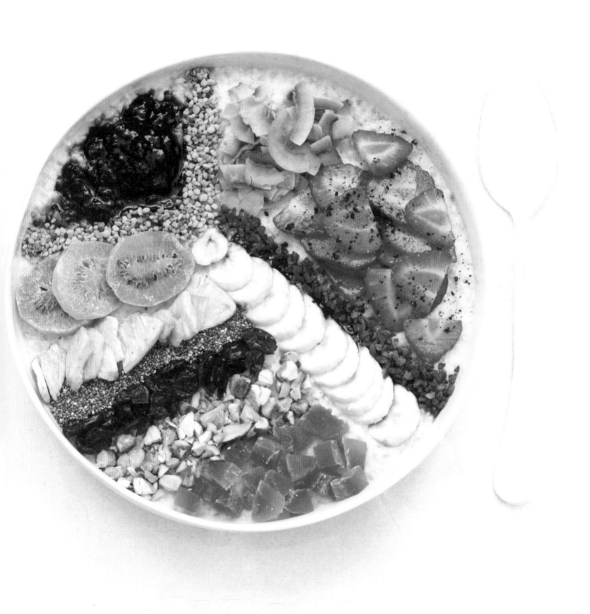

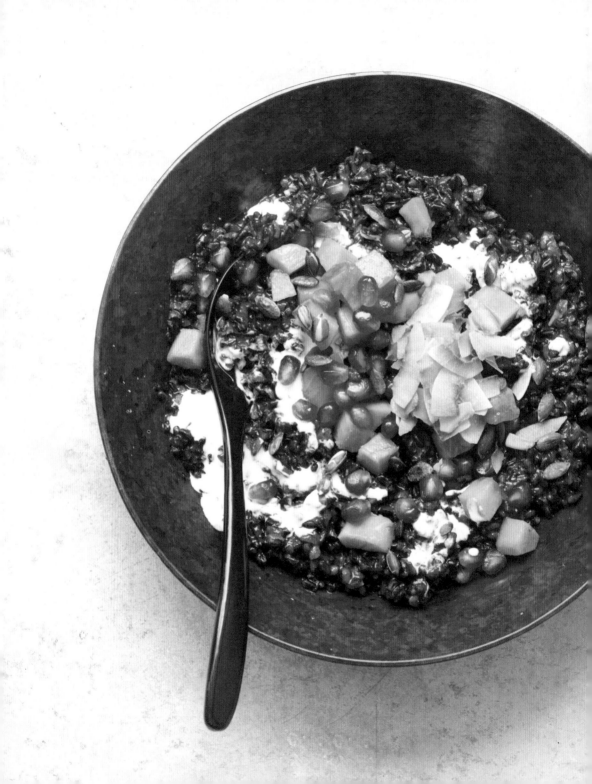

# CHAI-SPICED BLACK RICE PORRIDGE

AS YOU MIGHT GUESS FROM ITS STRIKING COLOUR, BLACK (SOMETIMES CALLED 'FORBIDDEN') RICE IS RICH IN ANTIOXIDANTS, AND HAS MORE PROTEIN, FIBRE, VITAMINS AND MINERALS THAN WHITE OR BROWN. IN COMBINATION WITH CHAI SPICES, IT MAKES A WARMING PORRIDGE.

**180 g/1 cup black 'forbidden' rice, soaked or rinsed**

**500 ml/2 cups water**

**250 ml/1 cup milk of choice (I like coconut), plus extra for serving**

**3–4 Medjool dates, stoned/pitted and roughly chopped**

**½ teaspoon vanilla powder or extract**

**½ teaspoon ground cinnamon**

**½ teaspoon ground ginger**

**¼ teaspoon ground cardamom**

**pinch of ground cloves**

**¼ teaspoon salt**

**OPTIONAL TOPPINGS**

**Toasted Coconut (page 29)**

**toasted pumpkin seeds/pepitas (page 30)**

**pomegranate seeds, mango slices or papaya cubes**

**SERVES 3–4**

In a medium saucepan, combine all the porridge ingredients together. Place over a medium-high heat and bring to the boil. Reduce to a simmer, cover with the lid slightly ajar and cook for 20–25 minutes, stirring occasionally, until the rice is tender and most of the liquid has been absorbed. Add a little more milk or water if you want the texture a little looser.

Serve with toppings of your choice and another little drizzle of milk.

# CARROT CAKE PORRIDGE

AT FIRST THE IDEA OF PUTTING GRATED CARROTS IN A SWEET PORRIDGE
SEEMED WEIRD, BUT THEY REALLY WORK HERE.

95 g/1 cup rolled/old-fashioned oats

375 ml/1½ cups water

250 ml/1 cup almond or coconut milk

2 carrots, grated

1 tablespoon pure maple syrup, plus
more as needed

2 teaspoons coconut oil

½ teaspoon pure vanilla extract

1 teaspoon ground cinnamon

½ teaspoon ground nutmeg

¼ teaspoon ground ginger

pinch of sea salt

1 teaspoon freshly squeezed
lemon juice

1–2 tablespoons almond butter
(optional)

**OPTIONAL TOPPINGS**

fresh coconut or coconut yogurt or
Coconut Whipped Cream (page 29)

(dark) raisins or sultanas/golden raisins

toasted walnuts (page 30)

SERVES 2

In a medium saucepan, combine all the porridge
ingredients, except the lemon juice, and place over
a medium-high heat. Bring everything to the boil with
the lid on but slightly ajar. Once boiling, reduce to a
simmer and cook for 10 minutes, stirring occasionally,
until the carrots are tender, the liquid is absorbed,
and you have a creamy texture. Stir in the lemon juice.

Stir in the almond butter (if using), then transfer to
bowls and serve with the suggested toppings.

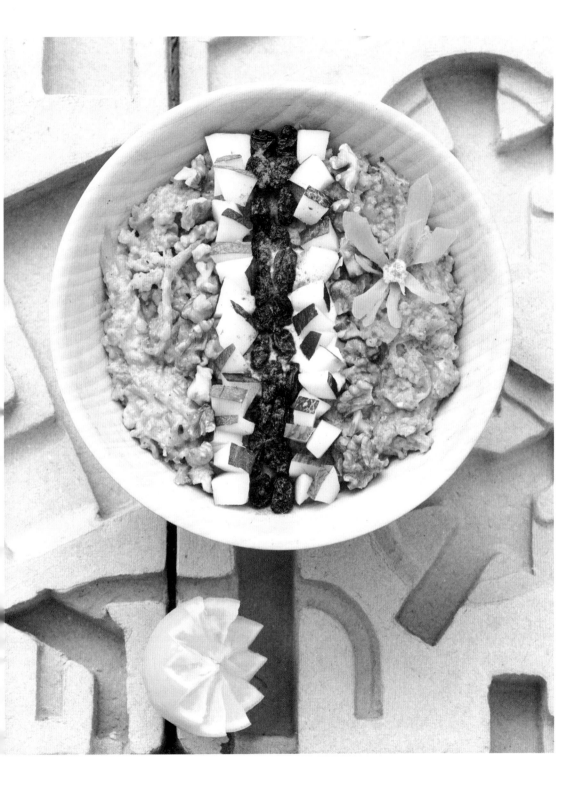

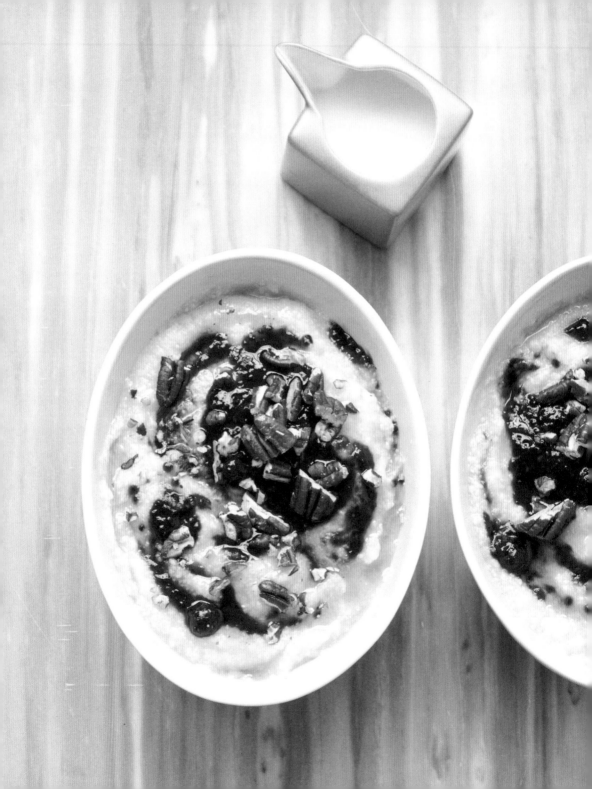

# BLUEBERRY MAPLE POLENTA

AS MOST GOOD PALS DO, ONE OF MY GIRLFRIENDS WAS RECOUNTING
A DELICIOUS BRUNCH OF CORNMEAL WAFFLES WITH BLUEBERRIES AND
MAPLE SYRUP. I INSTANTLY THOUGHT OF A SWEET POLENTA DISH WITH
A SIMILAR VIBE. IT'S SIMPLE, BUT THE FLAVOURS PLAY OFF EACH OTHER
SO NICELY AND THE COLOUR COMBO IS A WINNER, TOO — GOLDEN
CORN POLENTA WITH DEEP VIOLET BLUEBERRIES.

**625 ml/2½ cups water**

**75 g/½ cup fine polenta/cornmeal**

**½ teaspoon salt, or to taste**

**OPTIONAL TOPPINGS**

**Blueberry Compote (page 33)**

**pure maple syrup, to taste**

**milk of choice**

**toasted pecans (page 30)**

**SERVES 2**

In a medium saucepan, bring the water to the boil.
Once it's at a rolling boil, stir in the polenta/cornmeal
with a wooden spoon, then reduce to a simmer.
Season with the salt and cook, uncovered and stirring
regularly, until the liquid is absorbed. For fine
polenta/cornmeal, this can take as little as 1 minute,
or up to 10 minutes. Cover and leave to stand until
you're ready to serve.

Divide the polenta into bowls and serve topped with
blueberry compote, a little bit of maple syrup, milk
of your choice and some toasted pecans.

# PECAN BANANA BREAD PORRIDGE WITH CARAMELIZED BANANAS

I LOVE BANANA BREAD MADE WITH BUCKWHEAT FLOUR, SO NATURALLY BUCKWHEAT PORRIDGE WITH CARAMELIZED BANANAS IS AN IDEAL SWEET BREAKFAST TREAT.

**165 g/1 cup buckwheat groats, soaked (or cracked buckwheat cereal)**

**750 ml–1 litre/3–4 cups water or milk of choice (or a mixture of the two)**

**½ teaspoon ground cinnamon**

**¼ teaspoon vanilla paste or extract**

**¼ teaspoon ground nutmeg**

**salt, to taste**

**1 ripe banana, sliced**

**CARAMELIZED BANANAS**

**1 tablespoon coconut oil**

**pure maple syrup, to taste**

**1 ripe banana, sliced**

**OPTIONAL TOPPINGS**

**toasted pecans (page 30)**

SERVES 3–4

Combine the buckwheat groats, water or milk, cinnamon, vanilla, nutmeg and salt in a medium saucepan and bring to the boil. Reduce to just above a simmer and cook, covered with the lid slightly ajar, for 10 minutes. Add the banana and cook for another 5–10 minutes. Remove from the heat. Using a stick blender, blend for 30 seconds to achieve a creamier texture. Alternatively, process half the porridge in a regular blender until smooth, then transfer it back to the saucepan and stir to combine. If you are using cracked buckwheat cereal, then skip this latter processing step.

Meanwhile, for the caramelized bananas, heat the coconut oil in a frying pan/skillet over a medium heat until melted and warmed through. Add a splash of maple syrup and let it bubble and froth for a little bit (about 30 seconds). Add the sliced banana and cook for 2–4 minutes, then flip and cook for another couple of minutes, or until caramelized and golden.

Serve the caramelized bananas immediately over the cooked porridge and top with toasted pecans.

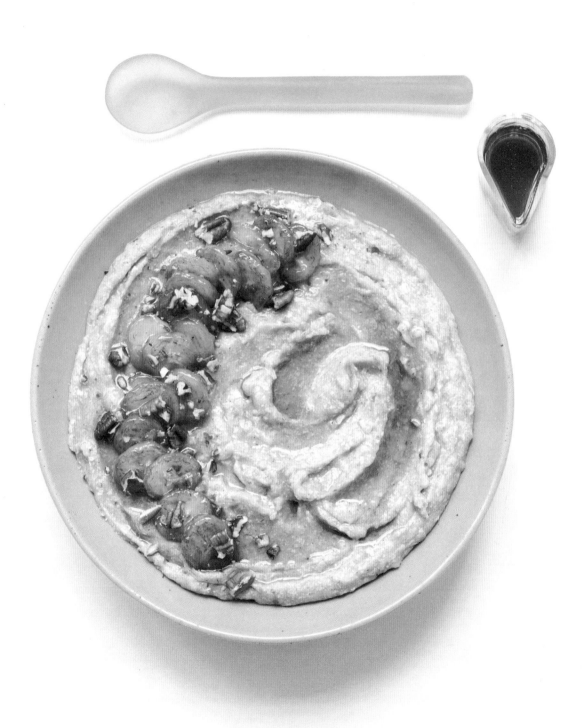

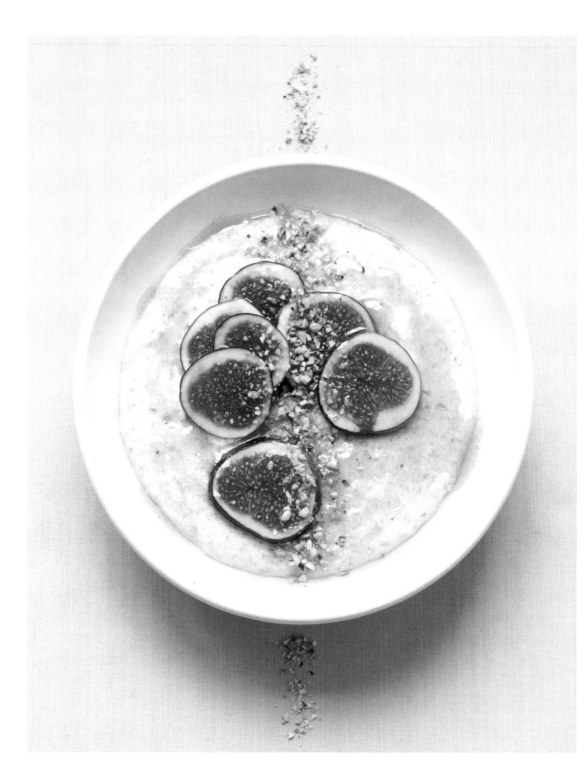

# RICOTTA, HONEY AND FIG PORRIDGE

RICOTTA AND HONEY ARE A MATCH MADE IN HEAVEN, AND IF FRESH FIGS ARE INVOLVED, EVEN BETTER. IF YOU CAN'T FIND FRESH FIGS, SWAP THEM FOR SLICED PEARS, NECTARINES OR BERRIES. YOU CAN USE TOASTED WALNUTS OR ALMONDS IN PLACE OF THE PISTACHIOS, TOO.

**95 g/1 cup rolled/old-fashioned oats**

**750 ml/3 cups water**

**½ teaspoon vanilla powder or paste**

**½ teaspoon ground cinnamon**

**55–110 g/¼–½ cup ricotta**

**OPTIONAL TOPPINGS**

**4 fresh figs, sliced**

**honey, to taste**

**2–3 tablespoons shelled pistachios, chopped**

SERVES 2–3

Combine the oats, water, vanilla and cinnamon in a pan. Bring to the boil, reduce to a simmer and partially cover with a lid. Cook for about 10–12 minutes, stirring occasionally, until the liquid has been absorbed.

When the oats are tender, remove the pan from the heat and stir in the ricotta. Divide between bowls and serve topped with sliced figs, honey and some chopped pistachios.

# PEACHES AND CREAM PORRIDGE

FRESH SUMMER PEACHES ARE ONE OF THE BEST SEASONAL TREATS.
CELEBRATE THEM WITH THIS PORRIDGE, TOPPED WITH COCONUT
WHIPPED CREAM FOR SOMETHING EXTRA SPECIAL. IF YOU EAT DAIRY,
YOU CAN SWAP THE COCONUT CREAM FOR DOUBLE/HEAVY CREAM.

**185 g/1 cup farro, soaked and drained**

**500 ml/2 cups water**

**250–500 ml/1–2 cups milk of choice**

**½ teaspoon vanilla paste or extract**

**¼ teaspoon ground nutmeg**

**pinch of sea salt, or to taste**

**2 teaspoons pure maple syrup, plus extra to taste**

**OPTIONAL TOPPINGS**

**2 ripe peaches, stoned/pitted and sliced into wedges**

**Coconut Whipped Cream (page 29)**

**toasted pecans or almonds (page 30)**

**blueberries**

SERVES 3–4

In a medium saucepan, combine the farro, water, milk, vanilla, nutmeg and a pinch of salt, and bring to the boil over a medium-high heat. Once boiling, cover with the lid slightly ajar, reduce the heat to medium-low and simmer, stirring occasionally, for about 30 minutes, until the farro is tender and creamy.

Stir in the maple syrup and taste for seasoning, adding more salt if needed. Add more liquid as needed for your ideal texture.

Meanwhile, if you haven't prepared your coconut whipped cream yet, go ahead and do that.

Portion the farro porridge into bowls and serve topped with the peaches and whipped cream, along with the other toppings, as desired.

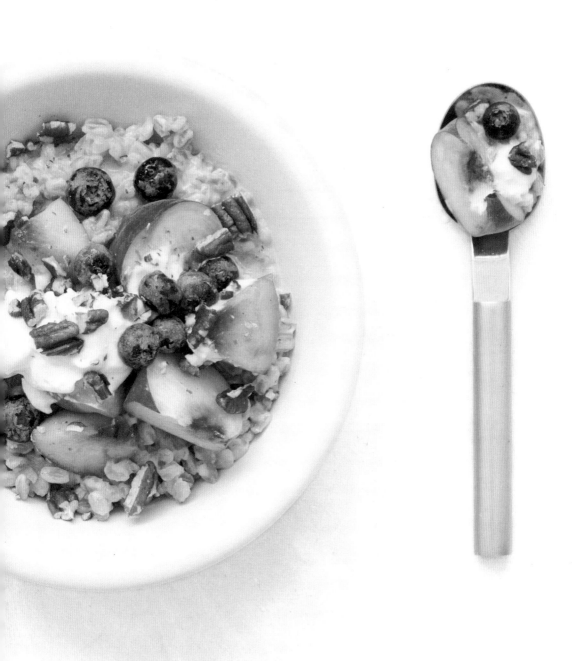

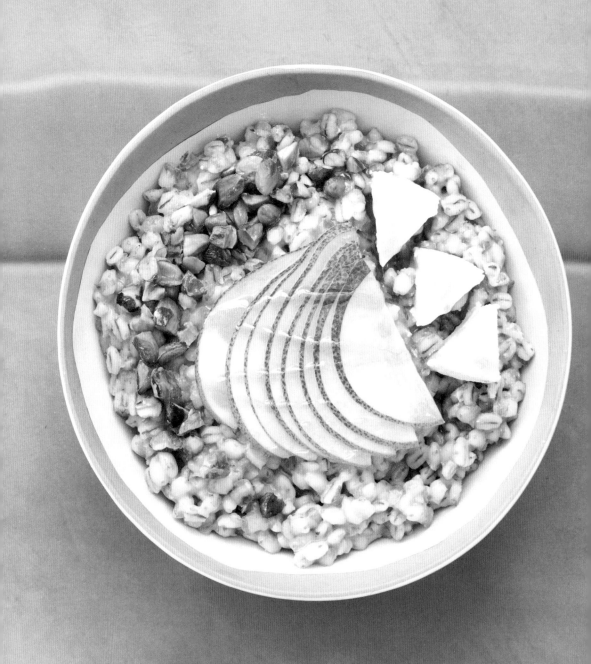

# PEAR, GOAT'S CHEESE AND HONEY PORRIDGE

THIS IS THE FANCY CHEESE PLATE OF PORRIDGES. GOAT'S CHEESE MAKES THIS BOWL POP WITH THE WINNING COMBINATION OF PEAR AND HONEY. FEEL FREE TO SUBSTITUTE PEAR FOR WHATEVER IS IN SEASON — SUCH AS PEACHES, APPLES, STRAWBERRIES OR FIGS. TO SPEED UP THE COOKING TIME, USE SOAKED COARSE OATMEAL/STEEL-CUT OATS OR ROLLED/OLD-FASHIONED OATS INSTEAD OF BARLEY.

**185 g/1 cup pearl barley, soaked and drained**

**750 ml/3 cups water**

**250 ml/1 cup milk of choice**

**pinch of salt, or to taste**

**½ teaspoon pure vanilla extract**

**1 teaspoon coconut oil**

**OPTIONAL TOPPINGS**

**1 ripe pear, halved, cored and thinly sliced**

**1–2 tablespoons crumbled or sliced goat's cheese per portion**

**honey, to taste**

**toasted pistachios or hazelnuts (page 30)**

**SERVES 3–4**

Combine the barley, water, milk, salt and vanilla in a medium saucepan and bring to the boil over a medium-high heat. Reduce the heat to medium-low, cover and simmer, stirring occasionally, for 40–50 minutes until the barley is tender. Towards the end of cooking, taste for seasoning, adding more salt if needed, and stir in the coconut oil.

Divide the barley porridge between bowls, add the toppings and serve.

# CINNAMON APPLE PORRIDGE

THE PERFECT COMBINATION FOR AUTUMN/FALL, THIS WARMING
PORRIDGE IS LIKE APPLE PIE IN A BOWL.

**185 g/1 cup farro, soaked and drained**

**750 ml/3 cups water**

**250 ml/1 cup milk of choice**

**1 teaspoon ground cinnamon**

**½ teaspoon pure vanilla extract**

**pinch of salt, or to taste**

**CINNAMON APPLES**

**coconut oil, as needed**

**1 medium-large firm eating apple, such
as Granny Smith or Pink Lady, cored
and cut into 1-cm/½-inch cubes**

**2 teaspoons freshly squeezed
lemon juice**

**125–250 ml/½–1 cup water**

**OPTIONAL TOPPINGS**

**pure maple syrup, to taste**

**Maple Pecan Granola (page 41)
or toasted walnuts (page 30)**

SERVES 3–4

First, break up the farro. Drain the soaked farro and
place it in a food processor or blender. Pulse for
30–60 seconds to break down the farro into smaller
pieces. This will help it cook quicker.

In a saucepan, combine the ground farro, water, milk,
½ teaspoon of the cinnamon, the vanilla and a pinch
of salt, and bring to the boil over a medium-high
heat. Reduce to a simmer, place a lid on and cook for
15–20 minutes, stirring occasionally, until thickened
and creamy. Taste for seasoning and add more salt
if needed.

Meanwhile, prepare the cinnamon apples. Heat
a large frying pan/skillet over a medium heat. Add
enough coconut oil to cover the base of the pan/
skillet in a thin layer when melted and allow that
to heat through for about 1 minute. Add the apple
cubes, lemon juice and the remaining cinnamon. Stir
to combine and cook for 1 minute. Add 125 ml/½ cup
of the water, cover and cook for 5 minutes, until the
apples are softened and sweet and the water has
mostly evaporated. If the pan gets dry before the
5 minutes are up, add a little more water.

Divide the warm farro between bowls. Top with the
cinnamon apples, maple syrup (if desired) and granola
or toasted walnuts.

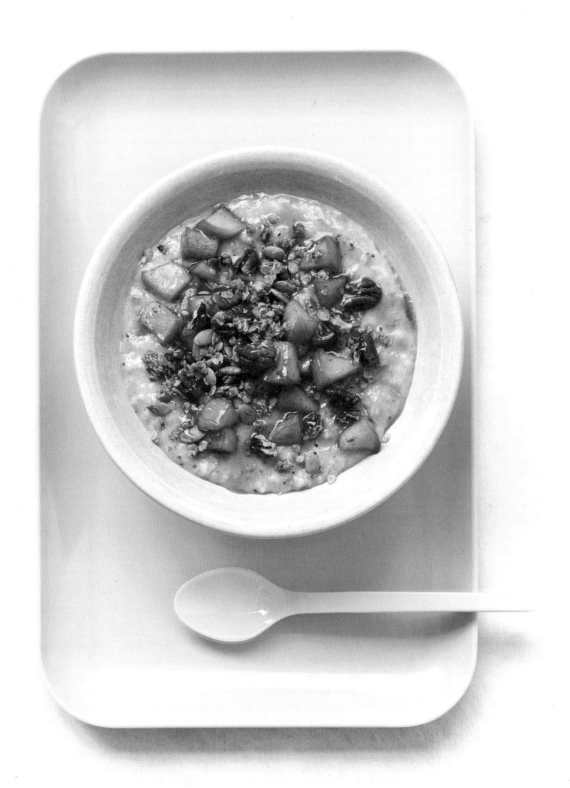

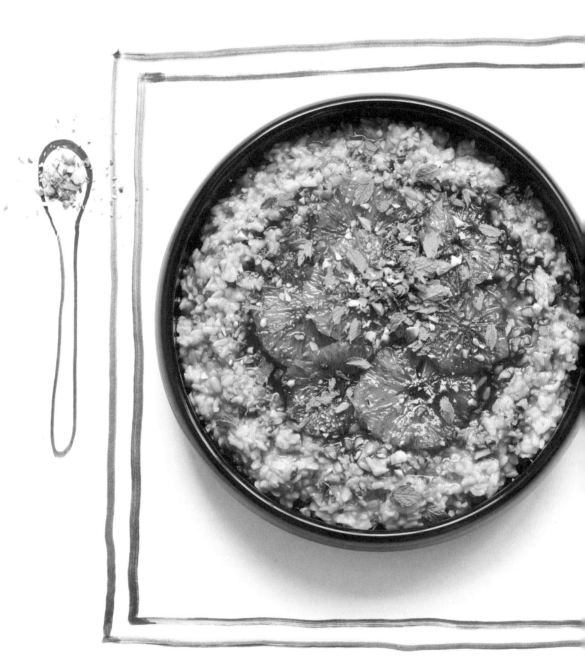

# EASY CITRUS BRÛLÉE PORRIDGE

I'VE FOUND THAT IN THE WINTER, CITRUS CAN REALLY LIFT YOUR MOOD
THANKS TO ITS COLOUR, TART SWEETNESS AND JUICY JOLT OF VITAMIN C.

**200 g/1 cup short grain brown rice, soaked and drained**

**750 ml/3 cups water**

**250 ml/1 cup milk of choice**

**generous pinch of salt, or to taste**

**1 teaspoon pure vanilla extract**

**½ teaspoon ground cinnamon**

**1 teaspoon coconut oil**

## GRAPEFRUIT

**1 large ruby red grapefruit, sliced into rounds, peel removed from the rounds (see Note)**

**2–4 tablespoons coconut or brown sugar**

## OPTIONAL TOPPINGS

**1–2 tablespoons finely chopped fresh mint**

**toasted pistachios (page 30)**

**honey (optional)**

*baking sheet, lined with foil*

SERVES 3–4

To cook the porridge, combine the rice with the water, milk, salt, vanilla and cinnamon in a medium saucepan. Bring to the boil, then cover with the lid slightly ajar, reduce to a simmer and cook, stirring occasionally, for 35–40 minutes. Once the rice is tender and the mixture is loose, but not too soupy, turn off the heat and leave it to stand for 5 minutes. Stir in the coconut oil, taste for seasoning and add more salt if needed.

Towards the end of your porridge cooking time, prepare the grapefruit. Preheat the grill/broiler on medium. Arrange the grapefruit rounds on the lined baking sheet, sprinkle each round with a layer of coconut or brown sugar and put under the grill/broiler for 5–7 minutes – watch it closely, making sure it doesn't burn. The sugar should be bubbling and caramelized. Remove from the grill/broiler and leave it to cool for a couple of minutes.

Serve the porridge topped with the brûléed grapefruit rounds, fresh mint, toasted pistachios and a drizzle of honey, if using.

Note: I find it's easier to slice grapefruit into rounds with the peel on, then remove the thin strip of peel from each round.

# NUTELLA-ISH PORRIDGE

THIS IS A PORRIDGE THAT PLAYS UP THE SIGNATURE FLAVOURS OF THE ITALIAN CHOCOLATE HAZELNUT SPREAD WITHOUT ACTUALLY ADDING ANY. BUT, IF YOU WANT TO ADD A DOLLOP, YOU HAVE MY BLESSING.

**90 g/½ cup ground buckwheat cereal (or untoasted buckwheat groats)**

**50 g/½ cup rolled/old-fashioned oats**

**pinch of salt, or to taste**

**375 ml/1½ cups water**

**250–375 ml/1–1½ cups coconut milk**

**2 tablespoons cacao powder**

**pure maple syrup, to taste**

**OPTIONAL ADD-IN**

**1 teaspoon maca powder**

**OPTIONAL TOPPINGS**

**1 ripe banana, sliced**

**hazelnuts, toasted and roughly chopped (page 30)**

**cacao nibs**

SERVES 2–3

Combine the buckwheat cereal (or groats), oats, salt, water and coconut milk in a medium saucepan and bring to the boil over a medium-high heat. Reduce to a simmer and, using a fork, whisk in the cacao powder and maca (if using) until incorporated with no clumps.

Cook, uncovered, for 10–15 minutes (if using whole buckwheat groats, it may take a little longer), stirring occasionally until creamy in texture. Stir in the maple syrup to taste.

When you are ready to serve, top the porridge with sliced banana, hazelnuts and cacao nibs.

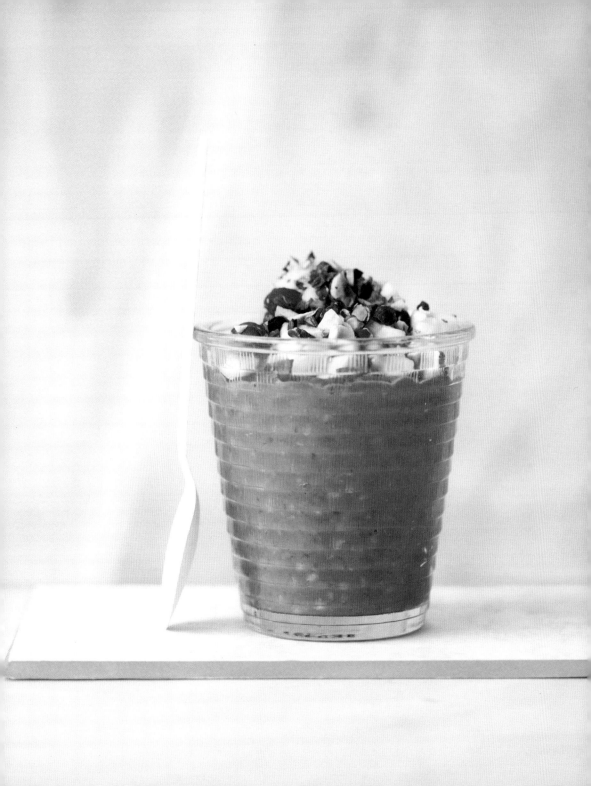

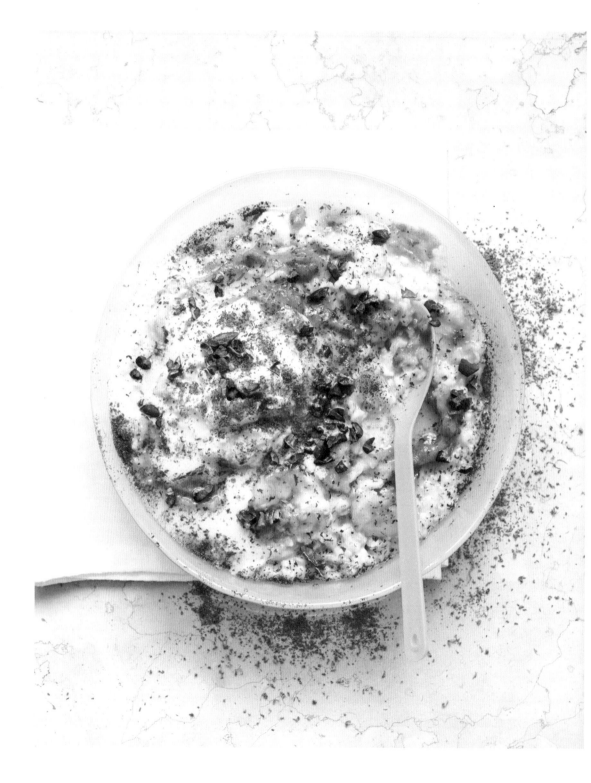

# BANOFFEE OATS

GROWING UP IN THE U.S., I WAS LATE TO THE BANOFFEE PIE GAME, BUT NOW IT'S UP THERE AMONG MY FAVOURITE DESSERTS. THIS IS THE PORRIDGE VERSION, AND OUR 'TOFFEE' COMES IN THE FORM OF DATES SIMPLY PURÉED WITH A LITTLE ALMOND BUTTER AND WATER.

**190 g/2 cups rolled/old-fashioned oats**

**1 litre/4 cups water (or a mixture of milk of choice and water)**

**pinch of sea salt**

**2 ripe bananas, sliced**

**DATE TOFFEE**

**10 dates, stoned/pitted and soaked in hot water for 5 minutes**

**3 tablespoons water, plus more as needed**

**1 tablespoon almond butter**

**pinch of sea salt**

**OPTIONAL TOPPINGS**

**Coconut Whipped Cream (page 29)**

**dark/bittersweet chocolate, grated on a microplane grater and/or cacao nibs**

SERVES 3–4

Combine the oats, liquid and salt in a medium saucepan over a medium-high heat. Bring to the boil, then reduce the heat to medium-low and simmer, stirring occasionally, until most of the liquid is absorbed; about 5 minutes. Add the bananas and cook for an additional 5 minutes until softened and sweet.

Meanwhile, make the date toffee by combining the dates and water in a food processor or blender. Process until a smooth-ish purée is formed, adding a little more water if needed. Add the almond butter and salt, and process again to incorporate.

Serve the porridge with a swirl of date toffee stirred in, topped with coconut whipped cream and grated chocolate and/or cacao nibs.

# PUMPKIN SPICE OATS

THE ULTIMATE AMERICAN AUTUMN/FALL STAPLE FOR THOSE WHO START CRAVING PUMPKIN PIE AROUND THE FIRST SEPTEMBER CHILL IN THE AIR.

**1 tablespoon coconut oil**

**1 teaspoon ground cinnamon**

**½ teaspoon ground ginger**

**¼ teaspoon ground allspice**

**¼ teaspoon ground cloves**

**¼ teaspoon ground nutmeg**

**pinch of sea salt, or to taste**

**140 g/1 cup coarse oatmeal/steel-cut oats**

**750 ml/3 cups water**

**250 ml/1 cup almond milk (or other milk of choice)**

**1 teaspoon pure vanilla extract**

**225 g/1 cup pumpkin purée**

**1–2 tablespoons pure maple syrup, to taste**

**OPTIONAL TOPPINGS**

**almond butter**

**toasted pecans or walnuts (page 30)**

**dried cranberries**

SERVES 4

Warm a medium saucepan over a medium heat and add the coconut oil. After the oil is warmed through and melted (about 1 minute), stir in the cinnamon, ginger, allspice, cloves, nutmeg and salt. Cook, stirring constantly, for 30 seconds until the spices are fragrant.

Stir in the oatmeal/oats to coat them in the oil and spices. Add the water, milk and vanilla to the pan and bring to the boil. Once boiling, reduce to a simmer, cover with the lid slightly ajar and cook, stirring often, for about 10 minutes.

Stir in the pumpkin purée and maple syrup, and simmer with the lid slightly ajar for another 20 minutes, stirring occasionally until creamy.

Serve topped with your choice of almond butter, toasted pecans or walnuts and dried cranberries.

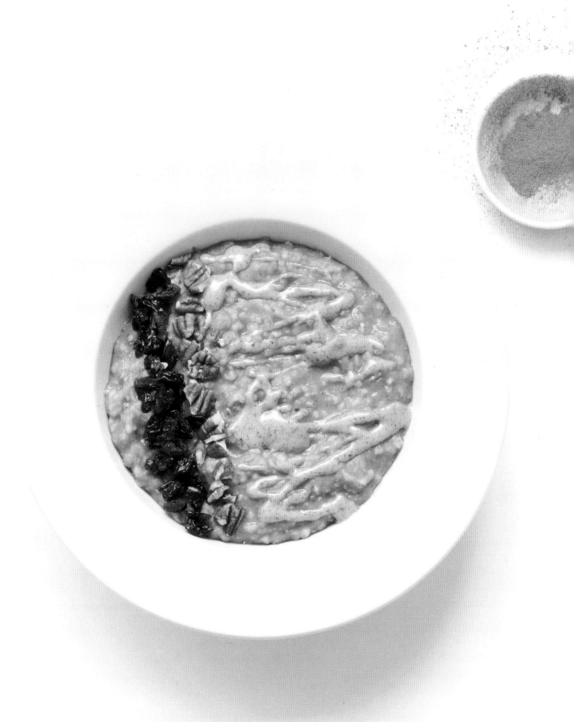

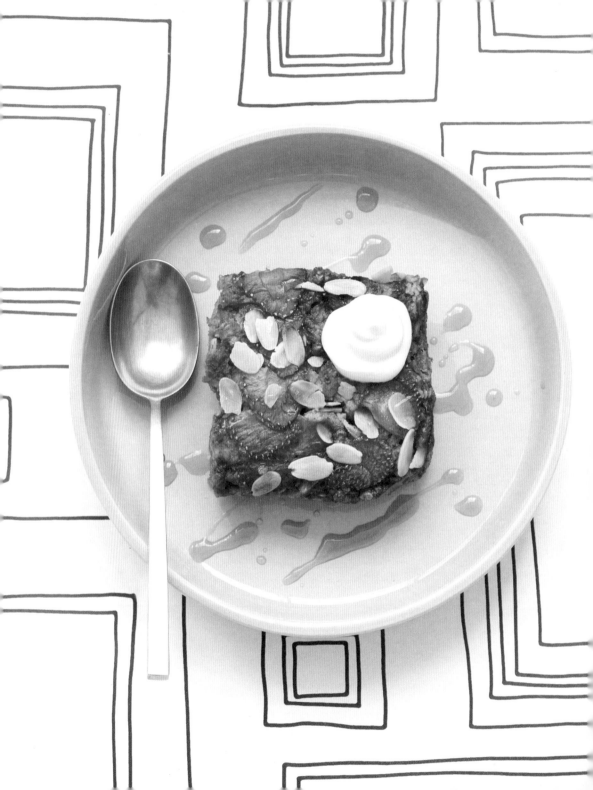

# BAKED PORRIDGE

*THIS IS GREAT FOR FEEDING BREAKFAST TO A CROWD OR FOR DOING YOUR FUTURE SELF A FAVOUR AND MAKING BREAKFAST FOR THE WEEK.*

**2 tablespoons ground chia seeds**

**6 tablespoons water**

**190 g/2 cups rolled/old-fashioned oats**

**50 g/½ cup ground almonds**

**2 teaspoons ground cinnamon**

**1 teaspoon baking powder**

**¼ teaspoon salt**

**2 ripe bananas, roughly chopped**

**375 ml/1½ cups milk of choice (I used almond)**

**60 ml/¼ cup pure maple syrup or honey**

**3 tablespoons melted coconut oil**

**2 teaspoons pure vanilla extract**

**450 g/1 lb. strawberries, sliced**

**60 g/¾ cup flaked/sliced almonds**

**TO SERVE**

**Greek-style yogurt or coconut yogurt**

**pure maple syrup (optional)**

*20-cm/8-inch square baking pan, greased with coconut oil*

SERVES 7–9

Preheat the oven to 190°C (375°F) Gas 5.

In a medium bowl, make a 'chia egg' mixture by mixing the chia seeds and water together. Let the mixture stand for 5 minutes.

In another medium bowl, combine the oats, ground almonds, cinnamon, baking powder and salt.

In the 'chia egg' bowl, mash the bananas with a fork. Add the milk, maple syrup or honey, coconut oil and vanilla. Mix well to combine.

Add the dry ingredients to the wet ingredients and stir to combine.

Add half of the sliced strawberries and 40 g/½ cup of the flaked/sliced almonds to the mixture, and pour everything evenly into the prepared baking pan.

Top with rows of the remaining strawberry slices and sprinkle the rest of the flaked/sliced almonds over the top. Bake in the preheated oven for 35–40 minutes until set. Cut into portions.

Serve warm or at room temperature with yogurt and more maple syrup, if you like it sweeter. Store in an airtight container in the fridge for up to 5 days.

# MILLET PORRIDGE
# WITH THYME-ROASTED PLUMS

I LOVE THIS IN THE LATE SUMMER WHEN I HAVE ACCESS TO A CRAZY AMOUNT OF PLUMS. WHILE THEY'RE GREAT AS IS, THEY ARE INCREDIBLE ROASTED. THE OPTIONAL STEP OF BREAKING UP THE MILLET IN A FOOD PROCESSOR REDUCES THE ALREADY QUICK COOKING TIME.

**200 g/1 cup millet grains**

**500 ml/2 cups almond milk (or other milk of choice)**

**500 ml/2 cups water**

**1 teaspoon pure vanilla extract or paste**

**pinch of sea salt, or to taste**

**2 teaspoons honey, or to taste**

**THYME-ROASTED PLUMS**

**2–3 firm plums, halved and stoned/pitted**

**1 tablespoon thyme leaves picked from stems, plus a few extra leaves to decorate**

*baking sheet lined with baking parchment*

SERVES 2–3

Optional step: Place the millet in a food processor, blender or clean coffee grinder, and pulse until it's just broken up, so that it is somewhere between flour and whole grain.

Put the millet, milk, water, vanilla and salt in a medium saucepan and place over a medium-high heat. Bring to the boil and, once bubbling, reduce the heat to medium-low. Simmer uncovered, stirring occasionally, for 15–20 minutes until creamy. Stir in the honey and taste for seasoning, adding extra salt if needed.

Meanwhile, preheat the oven to 190°C (375°F) Gas 5.

Place the plums, skin-side down (cut-side up), on the lined baking sheet, sprinkle the thyme leaves over and roast in the preheated oven for 10–15 minutes, until extra juicy and tender.

Serve bowls of millet porridge each topped with roasted plums and a few extra fresh thyme leaves to decorate.

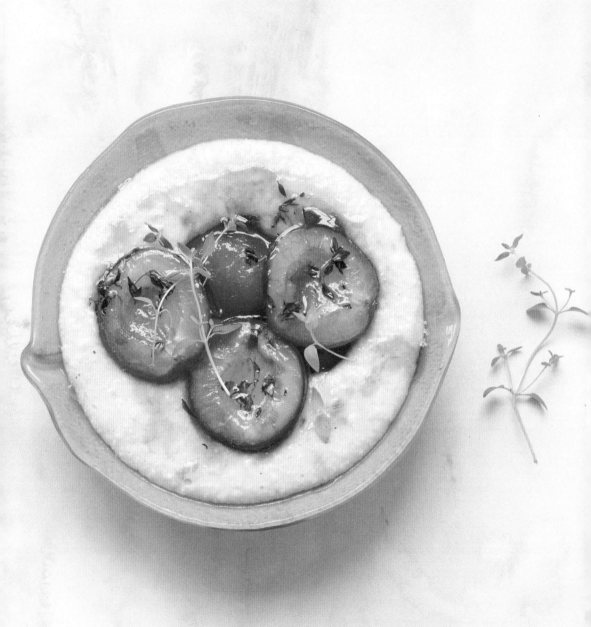

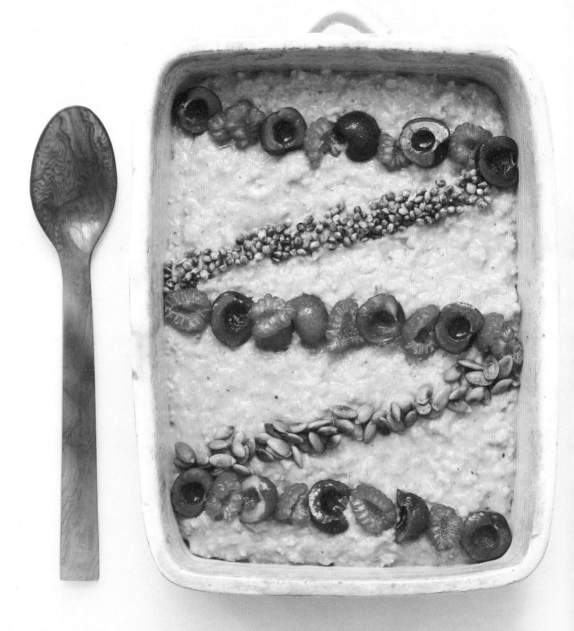

# GOLDEN PORRIDGE

INSPIRED BY GOLDEN MILK, THIS PORRIDGE IS A GREAT ANTI-
INFLAMMATORY WAY TO START YOUR DAY. I ADD A LITTLE BLACK PEPPER
HERE, WHICH (ALONG WITH SOME HEALTHY FAT FROM THE COCONUT
OIL OR GHEE) ACTUALLY HELPS YOUR BODY ABSORB THE TURMERIC.

**95 g/1 cup rolled/old-fashioned oats**

**250 ml/1 cup water**

**250 ml/1 cup almond milk (or other milk of choice)**

**½ teaspoon ground cinnamon**

**½ teaspoon ground turmeric**

**¼ teaspoon ground cardamom**

**¼ teaspoon freshly ground black pepper**

**pinch of sea salt, or to taste**

**1 ripe banana, sliced**

**1 teaspoon coconut oil or ghee**

**OPTIONAL TOPPINGS**

**raspberries**

**stoned/pitted cherries**

**hemp seeds**

**toasted pumpkin seeds/pepitas (page 30)**

SERVES 2

In a medium saucepan, combine the oats, water, milk, cinnamon, turmeric, cardamom, black pepper and salt, and bring to the boil over a medium-high heat. Once boiling, reduce the heat to medium-low and cook at a simmer for 5 minutes, stirring occasionally.

Add the banana and cook for another 5 minutes. Stir in the coconut oil or ghee.

Divide between bowls and serve with raspberries, cherries, hemp seeds and toasted pumpkin seeds/pepitas, as desired.

# SWEET POTATO PURÉE PORRIDGE

THIS PORRIDGE WAS BORN OUT OF MY LOVE FOR STARTING THE DAY WITH A BIG SERVING OF VEGETABLES, AND I FIND THIS PORRIDGE A SATISFYING OPTION ON A GREY DAY. I LOVE IT WITH FRESH BERRIES IF I HAVE THEM, OR DEFROSTED FROZEN RASPBERRIES OR BLUEBERRIES.

**1 large sweet potato (or 2 small), scrubbed clean and pricked with a fork a few times**

**500 ml/2 cups almond milk (or half almond milk, half water)**

**2 tablespoons chia seeds**

**2 tablespoons ground flax seeds/ linseeds**

**1 teaspoon ground cinnamon**

**¼ teaspoon ground cardamom**

**pinch of sea salt**

**1 teaspoon coconut oil**

**1–2 tablespoons almond butter**

**OPTIONAL TOPPINGS**

**sliced fresh berries**

**fresh edible flowers**

**Maple Pecan Granola (page 41)**

SERVES 2

The night before, preheat the oven to 200°C (400°F) Gas 6. Roast the sweet potato for 45 minutes until softened and cooked through (give it a little squeeze with a kitchen towel protecting your hands; if it has got a good amount of give, it's done). Leave it to cool completely, then store in the fridge overnight. You can do this in bigger batches for a double batch of porridge or for other meals.

In the morning, remove the skin from the sweet potato (it should peel away easily after it's roasted and cooled). Place it in a medium saucepan and mash it with a fork until you've created a rough purée.

Place the saucepan with the sweet potato over a medium heat. Stir in the milk, chia seeds, flax seeds/ linseeds, cinnamon, cardamom and salt. Cook, uncovered, stirring occasionally and further mashing the sweet potato as needed, for 5–6 minutes until the ingredients have warmed through and melded together in a thick but easily stirred consistency.

Stir in the coconut oil and either stir in the almond butter or drizzle it on with your other toppings.

Portion the porridge into bowls and serve warm topped with berries and granola.

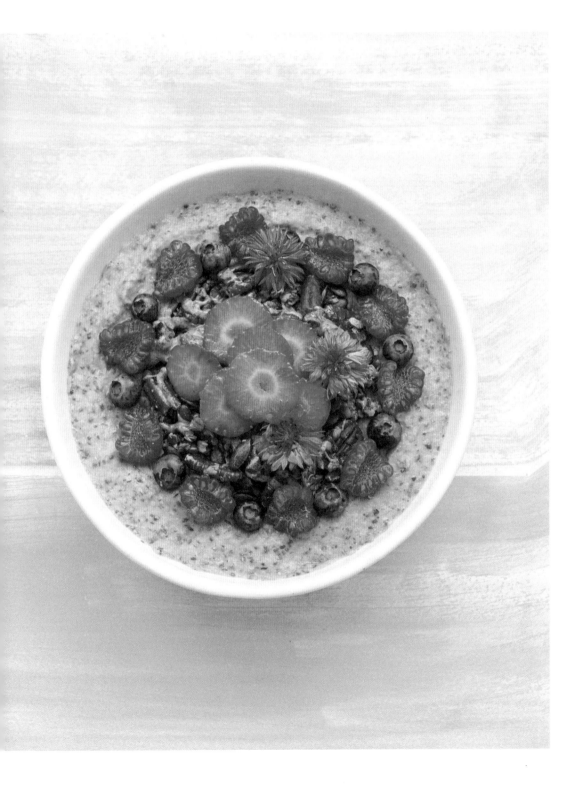

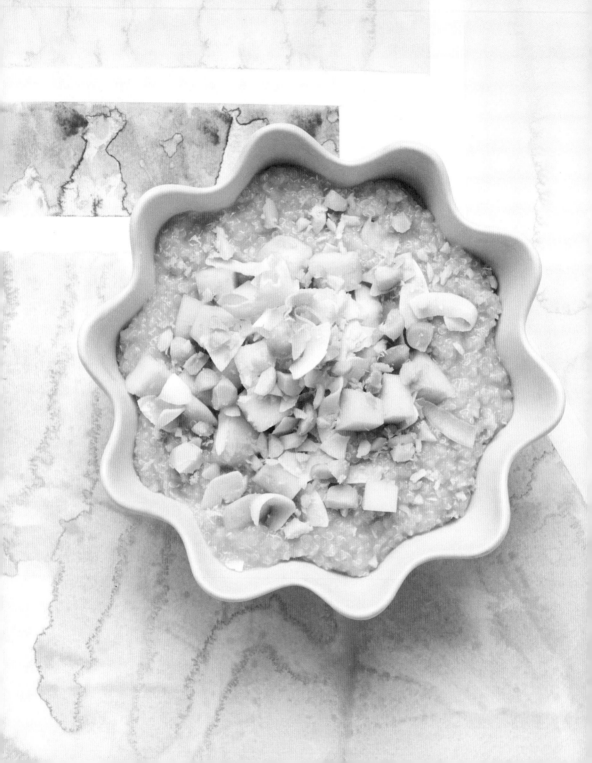

# COCONUT PORRIDGE AND MANGO

I THOUGHT I LIKED MANGOES UNTIL I MOVED TO AUSTRALIA... THEN
I REALIZED I LOVED THEM. WHILE A PERFECTLY RIPE MANGO DOESN'T
NEED ANY EMBELLISHMENT, THIS NUTTY COCONUT QUINOA IS A GREAT
COMPLEMENT FOR SWEET AND SUNNY MANGO CHUNKS.

**170 g/1 cup quinoa, rinsed**

**400-g/14-oz can coconut milk**

**1 teaspoon pure vanilla extract**

**pinch of sea salt**

**TOPPINGS**

**1 small-medium ripe mango,
peeled, stoned/pitted and cut into
bite-sized pieces**

**Toasted Coconut (page 29)**

**macadamias or cashews, lightly
toasted and roughly chopped
(page 30)**

**SERVES 2**

In a saucepan, combine the quinoa and coconut milk, then refill the coconut milk can with water (about 400 ml/1¾ cups) and add that to the saucepan, along with the vanilla and salt.

Bring everything to the boil over a medium-high heat, then reduce to a simmer and cook, uncovered, stirring frequently, for about 15 minutes until tender.

Serve the porridge with fresh mango pieces, toasted coconut and chopped nuts.

# RHUBARB CRUMBLE PORRIDGE

QUINOA AND AMARANTH ARE PART OF THE PSEUDOGRAINS FAMILY –
NUTRITIOUS SEEDS THAT ACT A LOT LIKE GRAINS.

**1 teaspoon coconut oil**

**85 g/½ cup quinoa, rinsed**

**95 g/½ cup amaranth, rinsed**

**375 ml/1½ cups almond milk (or other milk of choice)**

**500 ml/2 cups water**

**1 teaspoon pure vanilla extract**

**½ teaspoon sea salt**

**1–2 tablespoons almond butter, to taste**

**RHUBARB**

**3–4 sticks of rhubarb, roughly chopped (if on the thinner side, use 5)**

**250 ml/1 cup water**

**¼ teaspoon ground cinnamon**

**2 tablespoons honey**

**OPTIONAL TOPPINGS**

**Cardamom Tahini Granola (page 38)**

**Coconut Whipped Cream (page 29) or coconut milk (optional)**

SERVES 2–3

In a medium saucepan, heat the coconut oil over a medium-high heat. Add the quinoa and amaranth and cook, stirring, for 2–3 minutes to toast the (pseudo) grains. Add the milk and water, along with the vanilla and salt, and cook, covered, for 15 minutes, stirring occasionally. Once most of the liquid is absorbed and the grains are tender, stir in the almond butter.

Meanwhile, in another medium saucepan, combine the chopped rhubarb, water and cinnamon and cover. Bring the water to a simmer and cook over a medium heat for 5–6 minutes. Take the lid off and stir; the rhubarb should be starting to break down. Stir in the honey and reduce the heat to a low simmer for 2–3 minutes. Your rhubarb should be soft and falling apart, and there should be no excess water, just a thick compote.

Top the porridge with the rhubarb, granola and coconut whipped cream or coconut milk, and serve.

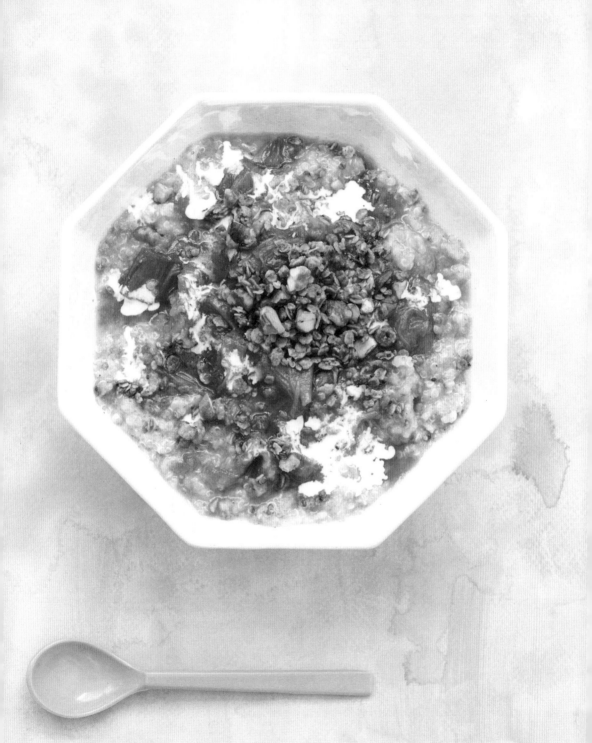

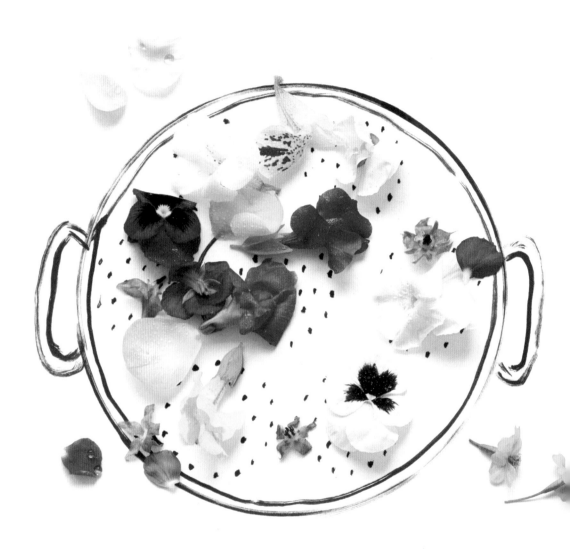

# COLD
## AND MAKE
# AHEAD

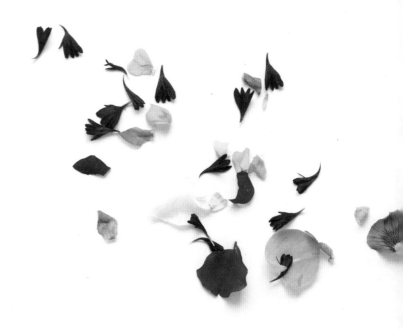

# CLASSIC BIRCHER MUESLI

CALL IT WHAT YOU WILL — OVERNIGHT OATS, OVERNIGHT PORRIDGE, ETC. — I CONSIDER IT BIRCHER MUESLI WHEN THERE'S GRATED APPLE INVOLVED. THIS IS PORRIDGE'S SUMMER OUTFIT, TO BE ENJOYED COLD WITH FRESH FRUIT AND A LITTLE YOGURT.

95 g/1 cup rolled/old-fashioned oats

1 tablespoon flax seeds/linseeds

¼ teaspoon ground cinnamon

pinch of salt

1 firm eating apple (such as Granny Smith, Pink Lady, or Honeycrisp), cored and grated, along with any juices

250 ml/1 cup almond or coconut milk (or half water, half milk of choice)

1 teaspoon freshly squeezed lemon juice

1 teaspoon pure maple syrup or honey

**TOPPINGS**
yogurt (Greek or coconut are great)

sliced fresh stone fruit – ideal when peaches, nectarines, apricots, and even cherries are in season – or try the Berry Compote on page 33

toasted flaked/sliced almonds

SERVES 2

Combine all the ingredients (except the toppings) together in a bowl and stir well to combine. Either cover the bowl or transfer to individual serving jars, and pop in the refrigerator overnight.

When you're ready to serve, top with 1 scoop of yogurt per serving, fruit and almonds.

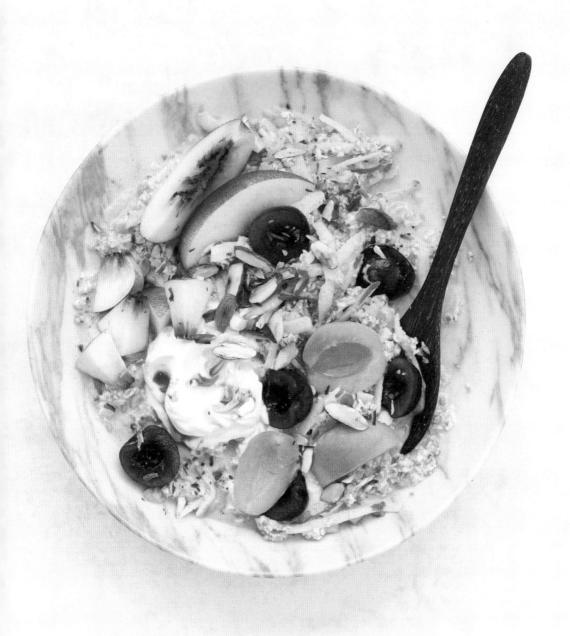

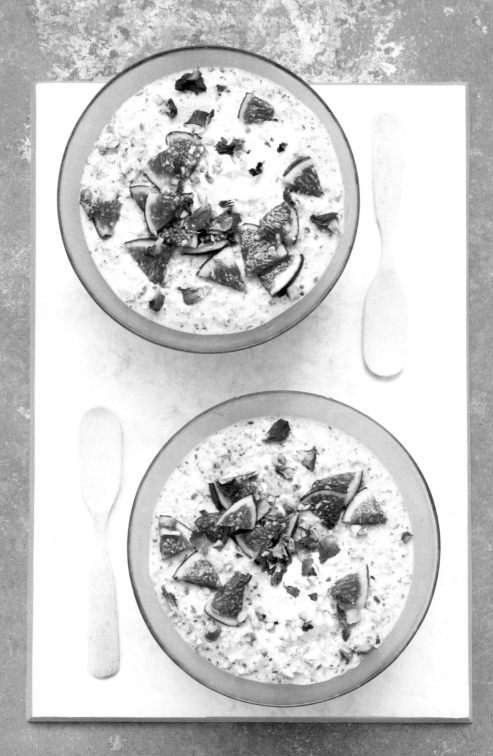

# ROSEWATER, PISTACHIO AND FIG OVERNIGHT OATS

IF FRESH FIGS AREN'T IN SEASON, CHOOSE SOME NICE RASPBERRIES
OR STRAWBERRIES INSTEAD. AND IF YOU'RE WORRIED THAT YOU WON'T
USE UP A BOTTLE OF ROSEWATER, LET ME REASSURE YOU. IT'S GREAT
IN HERBAL TEA AND STIRRED INTO SWEET DISHES SUCH AS THIS ONE,
BUT IT ALSO MAKES THE BEST FACIAL SPRAY/TONER. I POUR SOME
IN A SMALL SPRAY BOTTLE WITH A LITTLE WITCH HAZEL (3:1 ROSEWATER
TO WITCH HAZEL RATIO), AND SPRAY IT ON MY FACE IN THE MORNING
AFTER WASHING OR IN THE AFTERNOON WHEN I NEED A PICK-ME-UP.

**95 g/1 cup rolled/old-fashioned oats**

**2 tablespoons ground flax seeds/linseeds**

**pinch of ground cinnamon**

**pinch of salt**

**250 ml/1 cup almond milk (or other milk of choice)**

**2 teaspoons rosewater**

**1 tablespoon honey**

**TOPPINGS**
**yogurt (Greek or coconut are great)**

**2–4 fresh figs, chopped**

**shelled pistachios, roughly chopped**

SERVES 2

Combine the oats, flax seeds/linseeds, cinnamon and salt in a jar with a lid and mix together. Pour over the milk, rosewater and honey and stir. Pop the lid on and place in the refrigerator overnight.

When you are ready to serve, portion the oat mixture into bowls and top with yogurt, chopped figs (or berries) and pistachios.

# MATCHA COCONUT OATS

THE OVERNIGHT VERSION OF A MATCHA LATTE — CREAMY, SWEET AND
GREEN. FOR AN EXTRA PROTEIN BOOST, TRY IT WITH A LITTLE CASHEW
OR ALMOND BUTTER MIXED IN WITH THE BANANA.

**95 g/1 cup rolled/old-fashioned oats**

**2 tablespoons chia seeds**

**1 teaspoon culinary-grade matcha
powder**

**½ teaspoon ground cinnamon**

**pinch of sea salt**

**400-g/14-oz. can coconut milk**

**½ ripe banana, mashed**

**1 tablespoon freshly squeezed lemon
juice**

**½–1 tablespoon honey**

**OPTIONAL TOPPINGS**
**fresh or frozen fruit (I love it with
blackberries or mango chunks),
thawed if frozen**

**Toasted Coconut (page 29)**

**toasted almonds (page 30)**

**hemp seeds**

SERVES 2–3

Combine the oats, chia seeds, matcha powder,
cinnamon and sea salt in a medium mixing bowl.
Add the coconut milk and stir to combine. Add the
mashed banana, lemon juice and honey, then transfer
to a jar with a lid and place in the fridge overnight.

In the morning, serve with fresh or frozen and thawed
fruit, toasted coconut, toasted almonds and hemp
seeds, if wished.

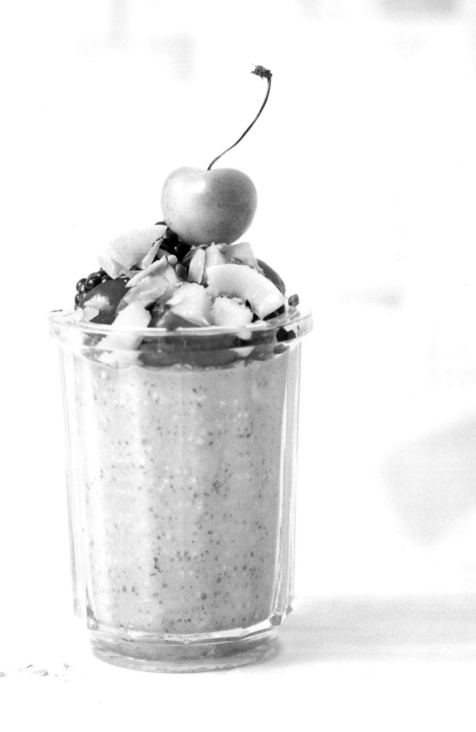

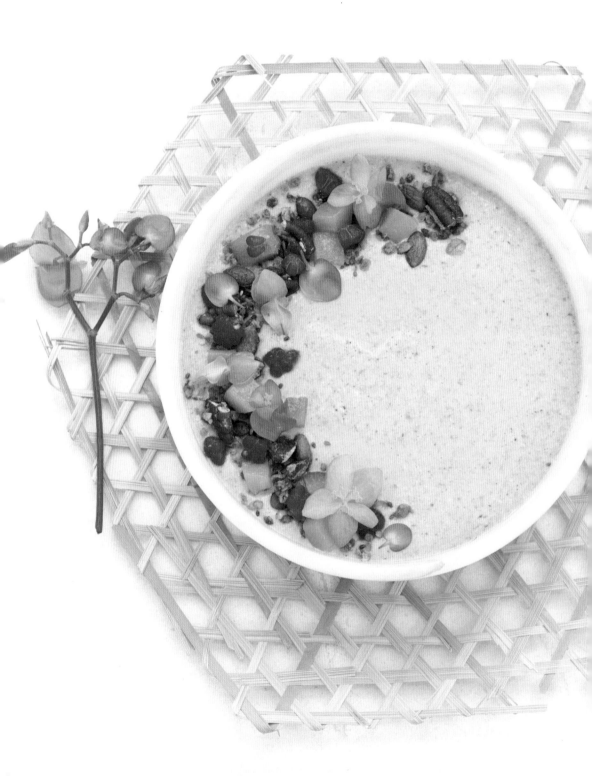

# RAW BUCKWHEAT AND BERRY PORRIDGE

THIS COLD PORRIDGE IS KIND OF LIKE A DAIRY-FREE FRUIT-FLAVOURED YOGURT. IT'S CREAMY AND SWEET, BUT IT'S ALSO PACKED WITH RAW SOAKED BUCKWHEAT THAT BRINGS LOTS OF FIBRE AND ESSENTIAL MINERALS SUCH AS MAGNESIUM TO THE MIX. SERVE AS YOU WOULD YOGURT — TOPPED WITH FRUIT, SUPER SEEDS AND CRUNCHY GRANOLA.

**165 g/1 cup raw buckwheat groats, soaked in water for at least 3 hours or overnight and drained**

**125 ml/½ cup almond or coconut milk**

**6–8 frozen strawberries (or 175 g/ 1 cup frozen raspberries)**

**¼ teaspoon pure vanilla extract**

**2 stoned/pitted dates, soaked in hot water for 5 minutes**

**1 tablespoon ground flax seeds/ linseeds**

**1 teaspoon maca powder (optional)**

**squeeze of fresh lemon juice**

**pinch of sea salt**

**OPTIONAL TOPPINGS**
**berries and diced mango**

**hemp seeds**

**fresh edible apple blossom**

**Maple Pecan Granola (page 41)**

SERVES 2

Place the soaked buckwheat and all the other porridge ingredients in a blender and process until the mixture is as smooth as possible, scraping down the sides with a silicone spatula from time to time, to make sure everything is well incorporated. Timing will depend on your particular blender, but this could take anywhere from 1–5 minutes blending time.

Serve with your chosen toppings. Store in jars in the refrigerator for up to 3 days, if desired.

# BLUEBERRY OVERNIGHT OAT SMOOTHIE

THIS IS A SMOOTHIE-OVERNIGHT OATS HYBRID, WITH THE BLENDED
BERRIES AND COCONUT MILK MIXED WITH THE OATS TO SOAK. DON'T
FORGET TO ADD THE HONEY (OR MAPLE SYRUP IF VEGAN), TO GIVE IT
THE RIGHT BALANCE OF SWEET AND TART.

**190 g/1 cup frozen blueberries**

**250 ml/1 cup coconut milk**

**1 tablespoon honey**

**pinch of salt**

**95 g/1 cup rolled/old-fashioned oats**

**1 tablespoon chia seeds**

**OPTIONAL TOPPINGS**
**toasted flaked/sliced almonds**
**or almond butter**

**fresh fruit, such as cherries,**
**blueberries or figs**

**sprinkling of dried blueberry powder**

SERVES 1–2

Combine the frozen blueberries, coconut milk, honey
and salt in a blender and process until smooth. In
a large jar with a lid, combine the oats and chia seeds.
Pour the blueberry milk mixture over the oats and stir
everything to combine. Pop the lid on and place
in the refrigerator overnight.

The next day, portion the oat smoothie into bowls
or jars, add the toppings and enjoy.

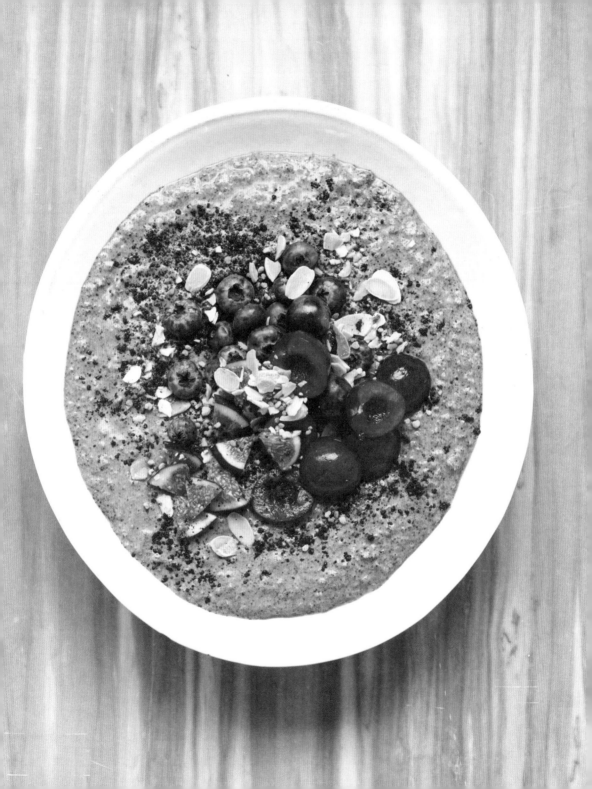

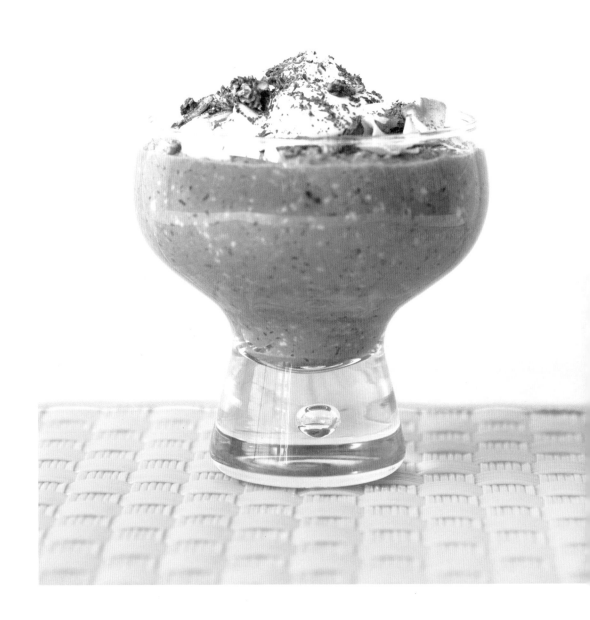

# TIRAMISU OVERNIGHT OAT PARFAIT

COFFEE AND CHOCOLATE IS A SOLID BREAKFAST COMBO. WHILE
THE TRADITIONAL ITALIAN DESSERT IS HARD TO BEAT, KICKING OFF YOUR
MORNING WITH THE OVERNIGHT OATS VERSION IS NEVER A BAD WAY
TO START THE DAY. I SAVE THE LEFTOVER COFFEE IN MY FRENCH PRESS
IN A JAR IN THE FRIDGE TO MAKE EITHER ICED COFFEE OR THIS RECIPE!

**95 g/1 cup rolled/old-fashioned oats**

**2 tablespoons ground flax seeds/
linseeds**

**2 tablespoons cacao powder**

**pinch of sea salt**

**125 ml/½ cup freshly brewed coffee,
cooled**

**125 ml/½ cup almond or coconut milk**

**1–2 tablespoons pure maple syrup**

**OPTIONAL TOPPINGS**
**Coconut Whipped Cream (page 29)
or plain Greek yogurt (see Note)**

**grated dark/bittersweet chocolate,
or cacao powder, or Chocolate and
Coconut Granola (page 37)**

SERVES 2

Combine the oats, flax seeds/linseeds, cacao powder
and sea salt in a jar with a lid and mix to combine.
Add the coffee, milk of choice and maple syrup, and
stir well. Pop the lid on and place in the refrigerator
overnight.

When you are ready to serve, top the parfait
with coconut cream or yogurt and grated chocolate
or cacao powder, or even some chocolate granola,
if you like.

Note: If using Greek yogurt, I'll sometimes stir a little
maple syrup into it before adding to my oats, for
a more dessert-like parfait.

# CHIA AND OAT PORRIDGE
# WITH STRAWBERRIES AND CREAM

THIS BASE IS A COMBO OF CHIA PUDDING AND OVERNIGHT OATS, AND
ITS SWEET VANILLA FLAVOUR PLAYS WELL WITH FRESH STRAWBERRIES
AND COCONUT CREAM. YOU COULD ALSO SWAP THE COCONUT CREAM
FOR VANILLA OR COCONUT YOGURT FOR A LITTLE MORE PROTEIN.

**4 tablespoons chia seeds**

**4 tablespoons rolled/old-fashioned oats**

**285 ml/1¼ cups coconut milk**

**½ teaspoon pure vanilla extract or paste**

**1–2 tablespoons pure maple syrup or honey**

**OPTIONAL TOPPINGS**
**fresh strawberries, sliced**

**Coconut Whipped Cream (page 29) (optional)**

SERVES 2

Combine the chia seeds and oats in a medium jar with a lid that's large enough to hold the liquid as well.

Combine the coconut milk, vanilla and maple syrup or honey in a bowl and whisk to combine. Pour the coconut milk mixture over the chia and oats and mix together. Pop the lid on and place in the refrigerator overnight.

Serve the chia and oat porridge with fresh strawberries and coconut cream (if desired).

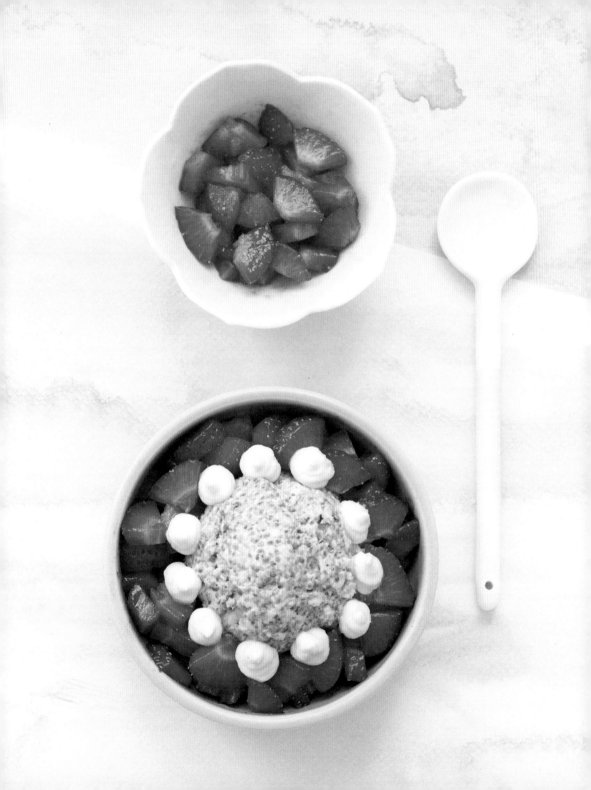

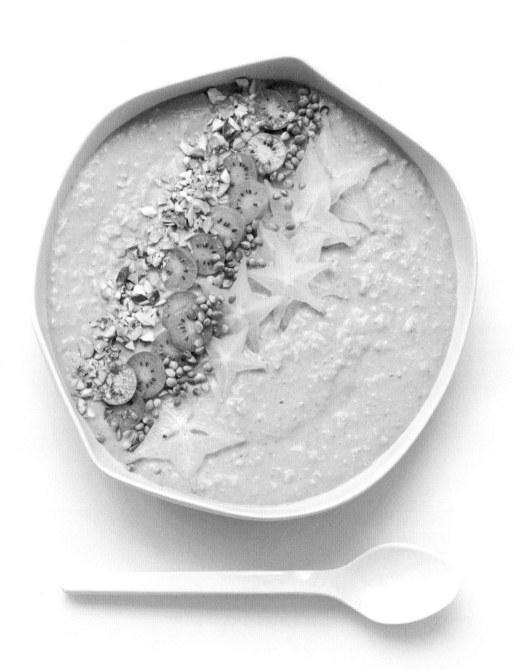

# BANANA AND SPINACH SMOOTHIE
# WITH CHIA OATS

THIS RECIPE IS A SMOOTHIE AND OVERNIGHT OAT HYBRID, THE SAME AS
THE BLUEBERRY SMOOTHIE ON PAGE 96 AND THE RASPBERRY VERSION
ON PAGE 108. REFRESHING, FILLING AND PACKED WITH ANTIOXIDANTS,
THESE ARE THE PERFECT SUMMER BREAKFASTS TO GRAB AND GO.

**1 frozen banana**

**155 g/1 cup frozen spinach**

**70 g/½ cup frozen pineapple**

**250 ml/1 cup coconut milk**

**¼–½ teaspoon spirulina powder (start
small, this stuff is powerful)**

**pinch of salt**

**95 g/1 cup rolled/old-fashioned oats**

**1 tablespoon chia seeds**

**OPTIONAL TOPPINGS**
**Toasted Coconut (page 29)**

**hemp seeds**

**sliced fresh fruit (such as star fruit
and kiwi)**

**roughly chopped pistachios**

SERVES 1–2

Combine the frozen banana, spinach and pineapple,
the coconut milk, spirulina and salt in a blender and
process until smooth. In a jar with a lid, combine the
oats and chia seeds. Pour the green smoothie over
the oats and stir everything to combine. Pop the lid
on and place in the refrigerator overnight.

The next day, portion the oat smoothie into bowls
or jars, add toppings and enjoy.

# CHOCOLATE PEANUT BUTTER CHIA POTS

COULD THIS BE A DESSERT? YES. BUT COULD YOU ALSO EAT THIS FOR BREAKFAST? YOU BET. CACAO IS GREAT FOR NATURAL ENERGY, HIGH IN ANTIOXIDANTS AND UNEQUIVOCALLY A HEALTH FOOD. HERE I COMBINE IT WITH CHIA AND PEANUT BUTTER FOR A PROTEIN-AND OMEGA-3-PACKED PORRIDGE-MEETS-PUDDING SITUATION.

**500 ml/2 cups coconut milk (see Note)**

**4 tablespoons cacao powder**

**3 tablespoons pure maple syrup, or extra to taste**

**3 tablespoons peanut butter, plus extra to serve**

**¼ teaspoon sea salt**

**80 g/½ cup chia seeds**

**OPTIONAL SUPERFOOD AND SUPERSPICE ADD-INS**
**1 teaspoon maca powder**

**½ teaspoon ashwagandha**

**1 teaspoon ground cinnamon**

**OPTIONAL TOPPINGS**
**fresh raspberries or strawberries**

**cacao nibs or dark/bittersweet chocolate chunks**

SERVES 4-6

Mix the coconut milk, cacao powder, maple syrup, peanut butter and salt (if you're using any superfoods or spices, add them now) together in a large bowl and blend with a whisk or a stick blender until you have a chocolate-y, peanut butter-y milk.

In a large jar with a lid, combine the chia seeds with the chocolate peanut butter smoothie, stir to combine, then cover and refrigerate overnight.

In the morning (or within a few hours), you'll have a thick, chocolate mousse-like mixture. Spoon into bowls or glasses to serve. Top with berries, a drizzle of peanut butter and some cacao nibs (or chocolate chunks!) to serve.

Note: Look for cans of organic, guar gum-free full-fat coconut milk (ideally, the only ingredients should be coconut and water). The texture can be thick, so I combine a 400-g/14-oz. can with 250 ml/1 cup of filtered water and keep it in a jar in my refrigerator to use throughout the week, or in a recipe such as this one.

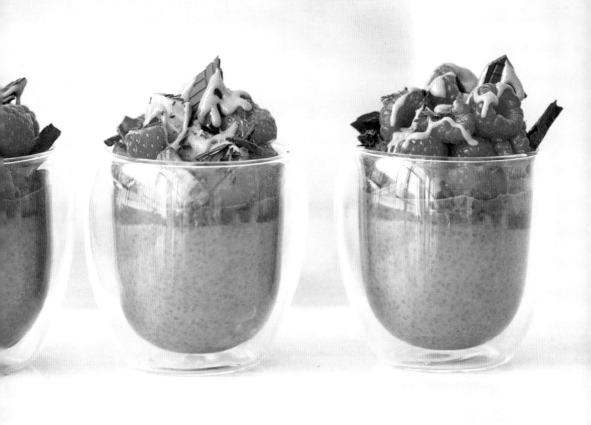

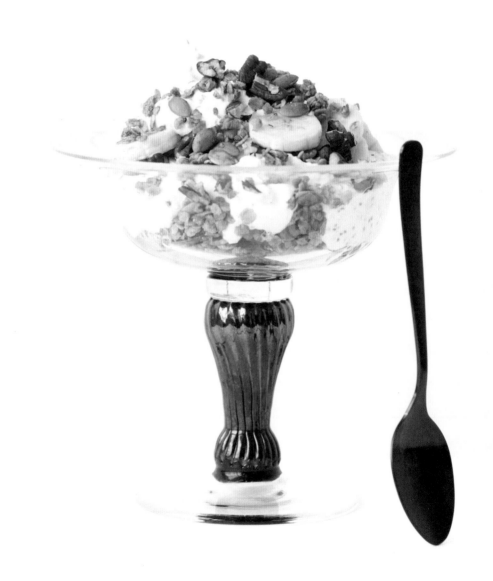

# BANANA CREAM PUDDING PARFAIT

NO SHAME: I HAPPILY EAT THESE CUPS FOR DESSERT AS WELL AS
BREAKFAST. THEY'RE SO SIMPLE, BUT GREATER THAN THE SUM OF
THEIR PARTS, AND IF YOU'RE A BANANA CREAM PIE OR PUDDING FAN,
I DEFINITELY RECOMMEND GIVING THESE A TRY.

**250 ml/1 cup coconut yogurt or full-fat plain Greek yogurt**

**¼ teaspoon pure vanilla extract**

**1 tablespoon chia seeds**

**pure maple syrup, to taste (optional: I usually only add maple syrup to Greek yogurt, as I find coconut yogurt is naturally very sweet)**

**60 g/½ cup Maple Pecan Granola (page 41) or Chocolate and Coconut Granola (page 37), or more as needed**

**1 banana, sliced**

SERVES 2–4

In a small mixing bowl, combine the yogurt with the vanilla extract, chia seeds and maple syrup (if using).

Divide some of the crumbled granola between the bases of two small jars or serving glasses (something with a 250-ml/1-cup capacity works well; if you're going for something more petite, try a 125-ml/½-cup capacity and split the mixture into four). Put a layer of the yogurt mixture on top, followed by a layer of banana slices. Top with more granola and repeat until the jars or glasses are filled. Place in the refrigerator until you're ready to eat and sprinkle more granola on top to serve.

# RASPBERRY SMOOTHIE WITH CHIA OATS

TEXTURE AND SWEETNESS IN A PRETTY SHADE OF PINK, THIS
COMBINATION OF SMOOTHIE, OATS AND CHIA PUDDING MAKES
FOR A TEXTURE-FILLED BREAKFAST THAT'S AS BEAUTIFUL AS
IT IS NUTRITIOUS.

150 g/1 cup frozen raspberries

250 ml/1 cup coconut milk

1 tablespoon pure maple syrup
or honey

pinch of salt

70 g/¾ cup rolled/old-fashioned oats

2 tablespoons chia seeds

**OPTIONAL TOPPINGS**
fresh fruit (such as redcurrants,
strawberries, pomegranate seeds,
peaches or nectarines, raspberries)

freeze dried raspberries

fresh edible flowers

nut butter (peanut or almond is great)

SERVES 1–2

Combine the frozen raspberries, coconut milk, maple syrup or honey and salt in a blender and process until smooth. In a jar with a lid, combine the oats and chia seeds. Pour the raspberry smoothie mixture over the oats and stir everything to combine. Pop the lid on and place in the refrigerator overnight.

The next day, portion the oat mixture into bowls or jars, add the toppings and enjoy.

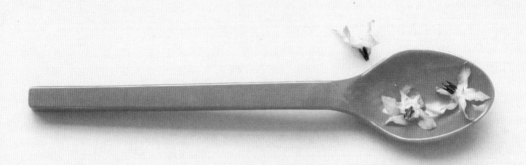
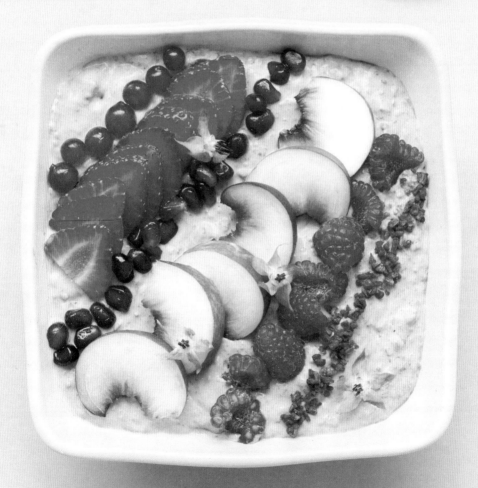

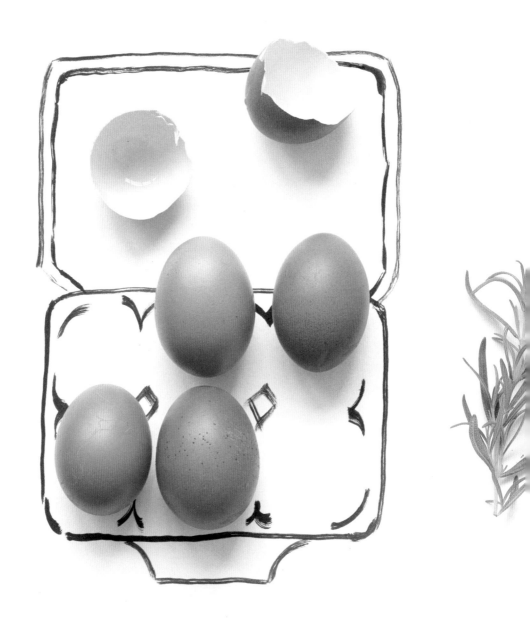

# SAVOURY
## AND COSY

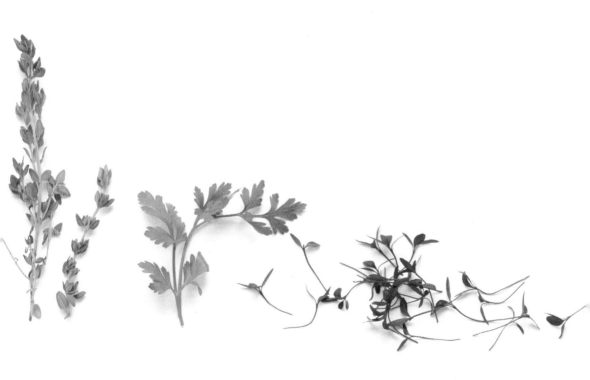

# FULL BREAKFAST PORRIDGE

NOT YOUR TYPICAL FRY UP, THIS VEGETARIAN BREAKFAST — COMPLETE
WITH MUSHROOM 'BACON' AND A FRIED EGG — IS SERVED ATOP
A BOWL OF QUINOA.

**85 g/½ cup quinoa, soaked for
at least 2 hours or overnight**

**375 ml/1½ cups vegetable, mushroom
or chicken stock**

**40–50 g/¼–½ cup Shiitake Mushroom
'Bacon' (page 45)**

**100 g/½ cup grape or cherry
tomatoes, sliced in half**

**1 big handful baby rocket/arugula,
spinach or kale**

**1 egg**

**sea salt and freshly ground
black pepper, to taste**

**olive oil or butter, for frying**

**OPTIONAL TOPPINGS**

**½ avocado, peeled, stoned/pitted
and sliced**

**your favourite hot sauce**

SERVES 1

Drain the quinoa and rinse. Put in a large saucepan
with the stock and bring to the boil. Reduce to
a simmer and cook, uncovered, for 15–20 minutes,
stirring occasionally, until most of the stock has been
absorbed but the mixture still has a loose, risotto-like
texture.

While the quinoa is cooking, you can prepare
the shiitake mushroom 'bacon' and other toppings.

In a medium frying pan/skillet, heat a little oil or
butter over a medium heat. Add the tomatoes and
a pinch of salt and cook for 5–6 minutes until softened
and golden. Remove from the pan and set aside.

To the same pan, add the rocket/arugula (or preferred
greens) and a pinch of salt and cook for 1–2 minutes
until wilted. Remove from the pan and set aside.

Wipe the pan clean with a paper towel, place back
over a high heat and add a little more oil or butter.
Crack the egg into the pan, then immediately turn the
heat down to low and cook for 3–5 minutes until the
white is just set and the edges are crispy. To help the
white set, I sometimes put a lid on the pan for
the last 2 minutes of cooking.

Once the quinoa is cooked, top with the tomatoes,
rocket/arugula, fried egg, and shiitake mushroom
'bacon'. Add some avo, a shake of hot sauce (I love
Cholula brand) and a grinding of black pepper, and
you're good to go.

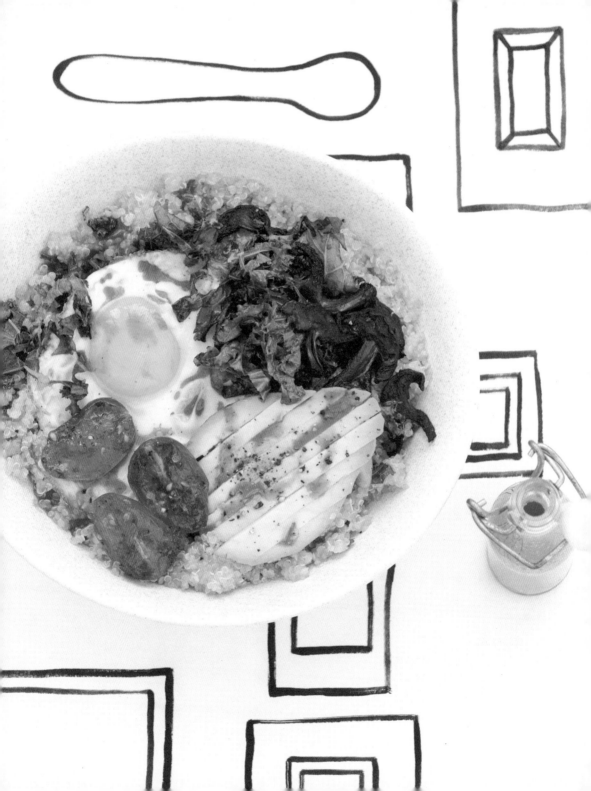

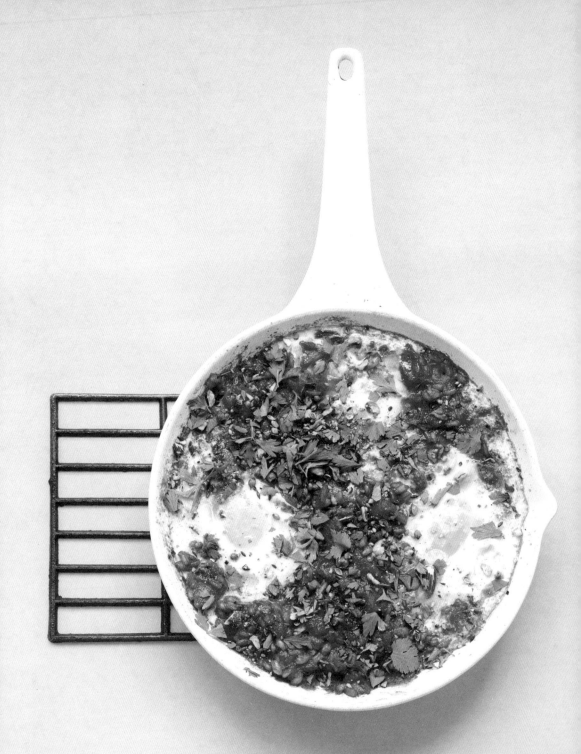

# SHAKSHUKA PORRIDGE WITH TOMATOES AND EGG

THIS GRAIN-BASED VERSION OF THE CLASSIC TOMATO AND EGG DISH HAS BECOME A FAVOURITE DINNER IN OUR HOUSE. IT'S FLAVOURFUL, SATISFYING AND LOVELY SERVED WITH A SIMPLE GREEN SALAD. IT CAN EVEN BE A ONE-PAN MEAL IF YOU SKIP TRANSFERRING TO A FRYING PAN/ SKILLET (WHICH I DO FOR AESTHETIC REASONS MAINLY).

**1 garlic clove, finely chopped**

**1 teaspoon ground cumin**

**½ teaspoon sweet smoked paprika**

**¼ teaspoon dried chilli flakes/hot red pepper flakes, plus extra to serve**

**185 g/1 cup pearled farro**

**400-g/14-oz. can chopped tomatoes**

**375 ml/1½ cups water**

**2–3 eggs, 1 per person**

**salt, to taste**

**olive oil, for frying and brushing**

## OPTIONAL TOPPINGS

**fresh coriander/cilantro and parsley, roughly chopped**

**Dukkah (page 30)**

SERVES 2–3

In a medium saucepan with a lid, heat enough olive oil to cover the base over a medium heat. Add the garlic, cumin, paprika and dried chilli/hot red pepper flakes and cook, stirring, for 1 minute. Add the farro, stirring to coat in the spices, then add the tomatoes, water, and salt to taste. Stir to combine and bring everything to a boil. Reduce to a simmer, cover, and cook for 20 minutes (depending on your farro, see Note below), stirring occasionally.

Once most of the liquid has been absorbed, transfer the mixture in an even layer to a lightly oiled medium frying pan/skillet and place over a medium-low heat. Make hollows in the farro mixture, crack the eggs into them, and cover. Cook for another 4–7 minutes until the egg whites are just set. Serve straight out of the pan (taking care with the hot pan handle), topped with fresh herbs and dukkah.

Note: Your farro may take a little longer if it's not pearled. Pearled grains mean that the bran has been removed, and this often speeds up cooking times.

# OAT PORRIDGE WITH SAGE-ROASTED BUTTERNUT AND CARAMELIZED ONION

THE COMPONENTS OF THIS BOWL MIGHT BE MORE LABOUR-INTENSIVE THAN WE'D LIKE FOR A TYPICAL WEEKDAY MORNING, SO I SUGGEST MAKING THE TOPPINGS AND PORRIDGE THE NIGHT BEFORE, OR ON THE WEEKEND. IN THE MORNING, JUST REHEAT AND ASSEMBLE.

1 quantity Classic Mixed Oatmeal Porridge (page 48)

3 tablespoons avocado oil (or other neutral oil)

2 large red onions, thinly sliced

1 tablespoon balsamic vinegar

pinch of dried chilli flakes/hot red pepper flakes, plus extra to taste

1 teaspoon honey

400 g/3 cups butternut squash (peeled weight), cut into 2.5-cm/1-inch cubes

1 tablespoon freshly chopped sage

salt and freshly ground black pepper

**OPTIONAL TOPPINGS**

finely grated Parmesan cheese

crispy sage leaves

extra virgin olive oil

*baking sheet lined with baking parchment*

SERVES 4

Prepare your oatmeal porridge (allow for overnight soaking time, if you haven't cooked it already).

Preheat the oven to 190°C (375°F) Gas 5.

In your largest frying pan/skillet, heat 2 tablespoons of the avocado oil over a medium heat. Add the sliced onions and a pinch of salt and stir to combine. Reduce the heat to medium-low. Cook for 15 minutes, stirring occasionally. If the pan gets too dry, add a small splash of water to keep things from sticking. Stir in the balsamic vinegar. Continue to cook for another 10–15 minutes, until the onions are softened, sweet and a little sticky. Remove from the heat and stir in the dried chilli flakes/hot red pepper flakes and honey.

Meanwhile, in a large bowl, toss the butternut squash cubes with the remaining avocado oil, the chopped sage and some salt and pepper. Spread out over the lined baking sheet. Bake in the preheated oven for 25–30 minutes, rotating the sheet after 15 minutes, until golden and tender.

If you prepared your squash and onions the night before, heat them through the next morning in a frying pan/skillet over a medium heat for 2–3 minutes.

Serve warm bowls of the porridge topped with the butternut squash and onions. Scatter with any additional toppings and enjoy.

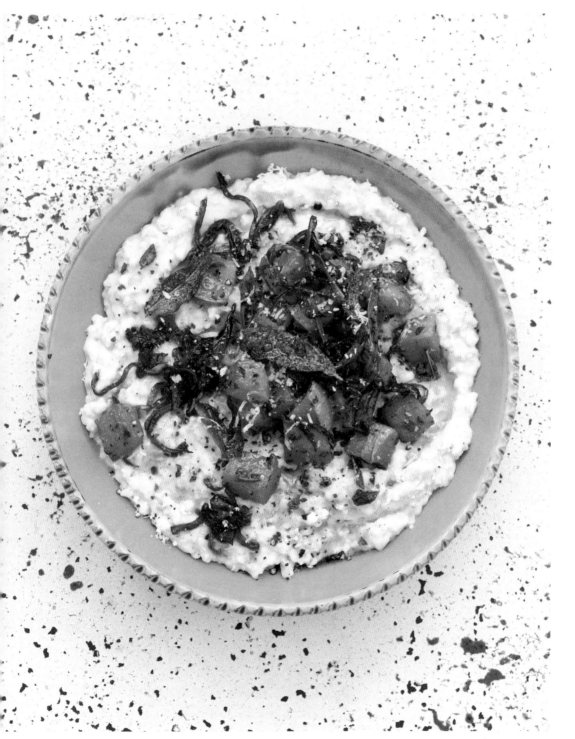

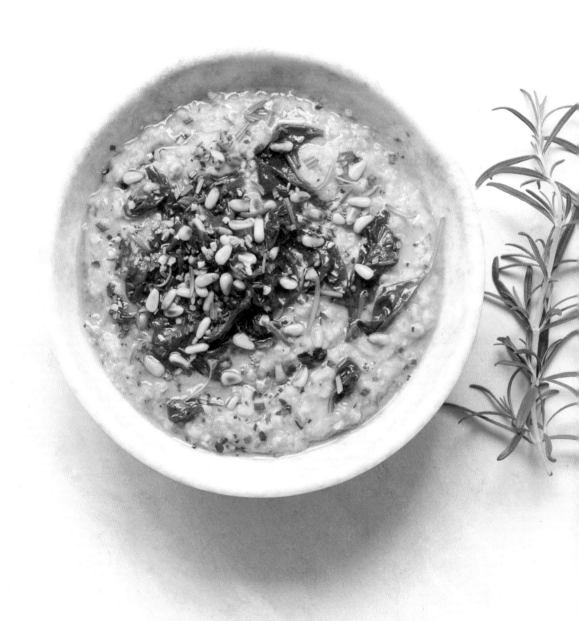

# CREAMY FARRO AND WHITE BEANS WITH ROSEMARY

COMFORTING AND PACKED WITH PROTEIN AND FIBRE, THIS CREAMY (BUT DAIRY-FREE!) DISH IS ONE THAT I'D HAPPILY EAT ANY TIME OF THE DAY. ROSEMARY IS A GREAT ADDITION TO THIS STEW-LIKE BOWL.

**3 garlic cloves, finely chopped**

**1 tablespoon freshly chopped rosemary leaves**

**90 g/½ cup farro, soaked and drained**

**500 ml/2 cups stock of choice**

**400-g/14-oz. can white beans, drained and rinsed**

**140 g/5 oz. baby spinach**

**dried chilli flakes/hot red pepper flakes, to taste**

**sea salt, to taste**

**olive oil, for frying**

**OPTIONAL TOPPINGS**

**toasted pine nuts**

**freshly squeezed lemon juice, to taste**

**extra chilli flakes/hot red pepper flakes**

SERVES 2–3

In a large saucepan, heat enough olive oil to coat the base of the saucepan over a medium heat. Add the garlic and rosemary and cook for 1 minute until fragrant. Add the farro and a generous pinch of salt and toss to coat in the aromatics. Pour in the stock, cover and bring to the boil. Cook, with the lid slightly ajar, stirring occasionally, for about 30 minutes or until tender. Stir in the white beans and cook for another 5 minutes.

Use a stick blender and blend for 30 seconds to partially purée the white beans and farro for a creamier texture.

Heat a medium pan or frying pan/skillet over a medium-high heat, add a drizzle of olive oil, the spinach, dried chilli flakes/hot red pepper flakes and a pinch of salt. Cook, stirring, until wilted, about 2 minutes. Taste for seasoning.

Serve bowls of the creamy farro topped with the sautéed spinach, toasted pine nuts and a squeeze of fresh lemon juice, to taste.

# MILLET GRITS WITH BBQ MUSHROOMS

A NOD TO THE SOUTHERN AMERICAN COMFORT FOOD FAVOURITE, SHRIMP AND GRITS, ONLY THIS TIME WE USE MINERAL-RICH MILLET AS OUR BASE AND MEATY MUSHROOMS GET THE BBQ TREATMENT.

**MILLET GRITS**

**200 g/1 cup dry millet grains, soaked and drained**

**1 litre/4 cups chicken or vegetable stock**

**salt, to taste**

**BBQ MUSHROOMS**

**½ teaspoon sweet smoked paprika**

**225 g/8 oz. mixed mushrooms including trumpet, cremini or king oyster, cleaned and thinly sliced**

**1 tablespoon barbecue sauce**

**1 tablespoon freshly chopped flat-leaf parsley**

**handful of baby rocket/arugula**

**avocado or olive oil, for frying**

SERVES 3–4

Combine the millet, stock and a pinch of salt in a large saucepan over a medium-high heat and bring to the boil. Reduce to a simmer and cook, uncovered, for about 15–20 minutes, stirring occasionally, until most of the liquid has been absorbed.

(Optional step) Take a stick blender and blitz the porridge for about 20–30 seconds to get a mix of creamy and textured millet. If the mixture is a little sticky or stodgy, add more stock or warm water and cook for an additional 5 minutes over a low heat. Allow to stand for 5 minutes.

While the millet is resting, prepare the mushrooms. In a large pan or frying pan/skillet, heat enough oil to cover the base over a medium-high heat. Add the smoked paprika, stirring it to combine with the oil. Add the mushrooms and cook for about 3–4 minutes, stirring only a couple of times until the mushrooms are seared and softened.

Once cooked, remove from the heat, season with a pinch of salt and stir in the barbecue sauce. Taste for seasoning. Divide the millet between bowls and top with mushrooms, parsley and rocket/arugula, allowing the warm porridge to slightly wilt the rocket/arugula.

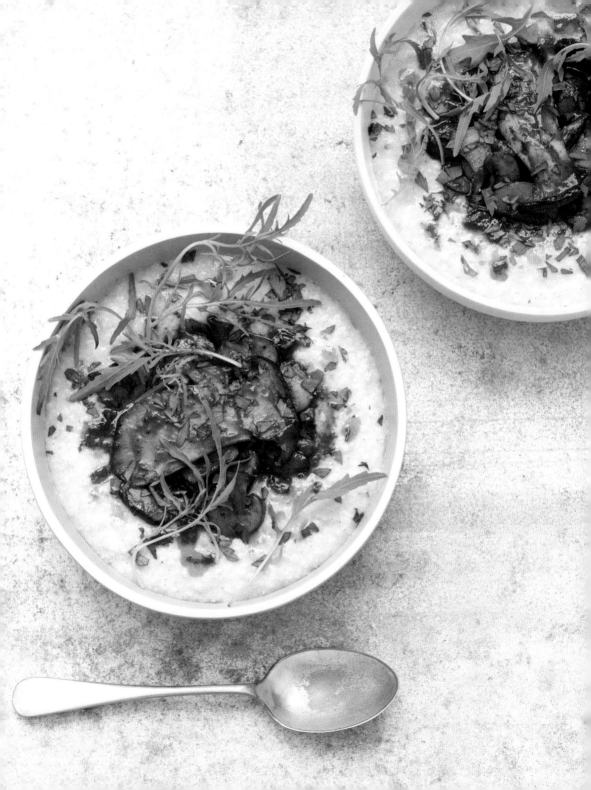

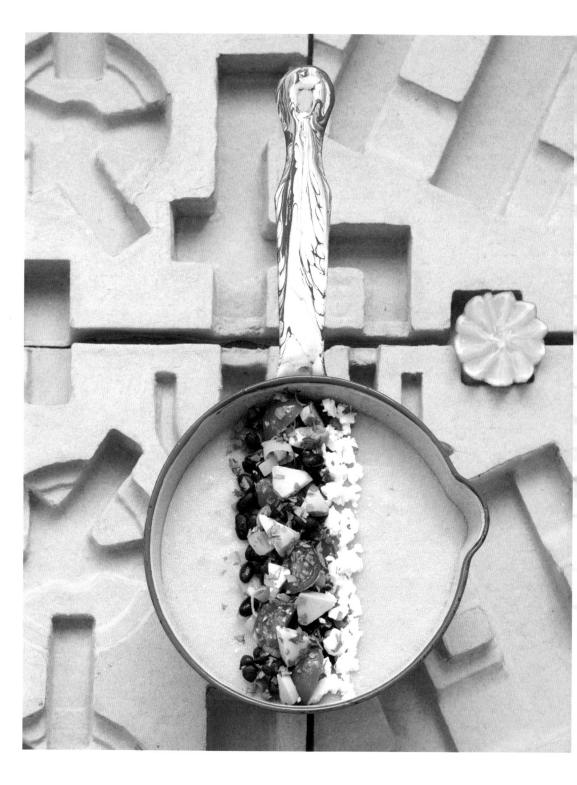

# MEXICAN POLENTA

THIS CORN-BASED POLENTA IS A GREAT FOIL FOR MEXICAN FLAVOURS,
BUT THE BLACK BEAN TOPPING IS ALSO GREAT IN TACOS AND SALADS.

1–1.2 litres/4–5 cups water,
or vegetable or chicken stock

150 g/1 cup fine polenta/cornmeal

3 spring onions/scallions, thinly sliced

225 g/8 oz. cherry tomatoes, cut into
quarters

2 garlic cloves, finely chopped

1 small jalapeño pepper, seeds and
pith removed, finely chopped

400-g/14-oz. can black beans, drained
and rinsed

freshly squeezed juice of 1 lime

salt, to taste

avocado or olive oil, for frying

**OPTIONAL TOPPINGS**

20 g/½ cup fresh coriander/cilantro,
roughly chopped

1 avocado, peeled, stoned/pitted and
cut into chunks

fresh cheese, such as Queso Fresco,
goat's cheese or feta cheese, crumbled

SERVES 4

In a large saucepan, bring the water or stock to the boil. Once boiling, stir in the polenta/cornmeal with a wooden spoon or silicone spatula, then reduce to a simmer. Season with a good amount of salt (I usually use around 1 teaspoon to start, depending on the liquid I'm using). Cook, uncovered, stirring regularly, until the liquid is absorbed. For finely-ground polenta/cornmeal, this can take as little as 1 minute, or up to 10 minutes. Cover and leave to stand until you're ready to serve. Note: If you've let it sit for a little while, you may need to gently reheat before serving and add a little more liquid to get it back to your desired consistency.

Meanwhile, in a large frying pan/skillet, heat enough avocado or olive oil to cover the base of the pan over a medium-high heat. Add the spring onions/scallions and cook, stirring, for 2 minutes. Add the quartered tomatoes, garlic, jalapeño and salt, to taste. Cook, stirring, for 2–3 minutes until the garlic is fragrant and the tomatoes are just softened. Stir in the black beans and warm through, about 1–2 minutes. Remove from the heat and stir in a spritz of fresh lime juice. Taste for seasoning, adding more salt or lime as needed.

Portion the warm polenta into bowls and top with the tomato/black bean salsa, coriander/cilantro, avocado and fresh cheese.

# LENTIL DHAL WITH GARLIC YOGURT

BECAUSE IT IS COMFORTING AND NOURISHING, THIS LENTIL STEW CAN
BE LIKENED TO A PORRIDGE AND ENJOYED AT ANY TIME OF THE DAY.

2 tablespoons coconut oil or ghee

1 medium onion, thinly sliced

1 teaspoon salt, plus extra to taste

2 garlic cloves, finely chopped

1 teaspoon grated fresh ginger

2 teaspoons ground cumin

1 teaspoon ground turmeric

1 teaspoon ground coriander

½ teaspoon garam masala

¼ teaspoon cayenne pepper

400-g/14-oz. can passata/puréed
tomatoes

270 g/1½ cups dried red lentils,
soaked, then drained and rinsed

2 carrots, finely diced

freshly ground black pepper, to taste

## OPTIONAL TOPPINGS

215 g/1 cup Greek yogurt mixed with
1 grated garlic clove and salt to taste

fresh coriander/cilantro leaves

Dukkah (page 30) mixed with dried
chilli flakes/hot red pepper flakes

SERVES 4–6

Heat the coconut oil or ghee in a large pan over
a medium-high heat. Add the onion and salt and cook
for 10–12 minutes, stirring occasionally, until softened
and starting to turn golden. Add a splash or two of
water if the pan begins to get dry. Add the garlic and
ginger and cook for 1 minute. Stir in the spices and
cook for 1 minute. Add the tomatoes and cook until
it begins to bubble again, then add 750 ml/3 cups
of water and the lentils and bring to the boil. Add the
carrots and reduce to a simmer. Cover and cook for
about 20 minutes, stirring occasionally, until the lentils
are broken down and creamy and the carrots are
tender. Check for seasoning, stirring in salt and black
pepper to taste.

Serve the dhal in bowls topped with the garlic yogurt
and any/all of the suggested toppings.

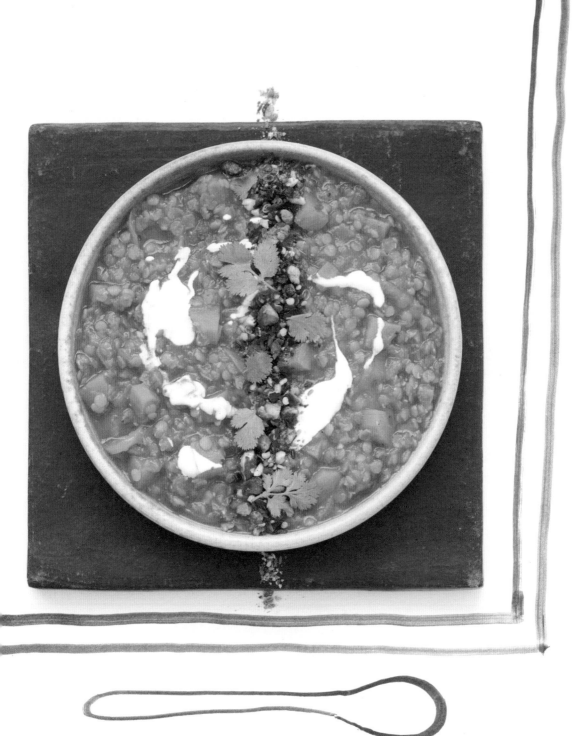

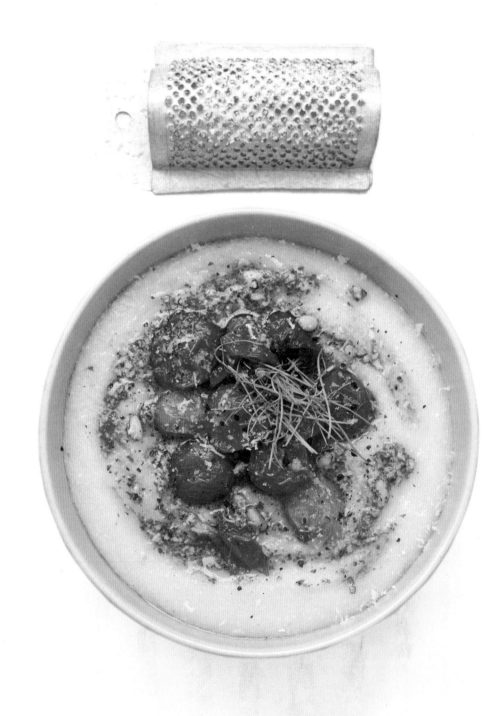

# ITALIAN POLENTA

THIS RECIPE DOUBLES AS A SAVOURY BREAKFAST OR EASY WEEKNIGHT DINNER. YOU CAN MAKE YOUR OWN PESTO IF YOU HAVE THE TIME AND PLENTY OF BASIL (SEE RECIPE ON PAGE 42) OR JUST USE YOUR FAVOURITE STORE-BOUGHT BRAND.

**350 g/12 oz. cherry or grape tomatoes**

**2 tablespoons olive oil**

**1.2 litres/4–5 cups water or stock of choice**

**150 g/1 cup fine polenta/cornmeal (the fine grind makes it cook very quickly!)**

**2 tablespoons finely grated Parmesan, plus extra to serve**

**sea salt and freshly ground black pepper, to taste**

**OPTIONAL TOPPINGS**

**4 tablespoons Green Pesto (page 42)**

**garlic chives (optional)**

*baking sheet lined with baking parchment*

SERVES 4

Preheat the oven to 190°C (375°F) Gas 5.

Spread the tomatoes over the lined baking sheet, sprinkle with a little salt and roast in the preheated oven for 15–20 minutes until collapsing and lightly browned in places. When you remove them from the oven, drizzle with 1 tablespoon of the olive oil and toss to coat. Taste for seasoning and set aside.

Meanwhile, in a large saucepan, bring the water or stock to a boil (if using water, you can boil it in the kettle first to save time). Once it's at a rolling boil, stir in the polenta/cornmeal with a wooden spoon, then reduce to a simmer.

Season with a good amount of salt (I usually use around 1 teaspoon, depending on the liquid I'm using). Cook, uncovered, stirring regularly, until the liquid is absorbed. For finely ground polenta, this can take as little as 1 minute, or up to 10 minutes. Cover and leave to stand until you're ready to serve. Note: If you've let it sit for a little while, you may need to gently reheat and add a little more liquid to get it to your desired consistency. Stir in the remaining tablespoon of olive oil, 2 tablespoons of Parmesan and a few grinds of black pepper.

Portion into bowls and top with a spoonful of pesto, roasted tomatoes, garlic chives (if using) and a sprinkling of Parmesan.

# BAKED EGG PORRIDGE WITH MUSHROOMS

THIS FRYING PAN/SKILLET-BAKED PORRIDGE IS A LITTLE MORE INVOLVED, BUT WORTH IT FOR ONE OF THE ULTIMATE HEARTY BREAKFASTS.

**70 g/½ cup coarse oatmeal/ steel-cut oats, soaked and drained**

**350 ml/scant 1½ cups boiling water**

**280 g/10 oz. mushrooms, sliced**

**1 tablespoon fresh thyme leaves, plus extra to garnish**

**55 g/¼ cup ricotta**

**2 eggs**

**salt and freshly ground black pepper, to taste**

**grass-fed butter or olive oil, for frying**

*small, ovenproof frying pan/skillet or baking dish, well-greased with butter or olive oil*

SERVES 2

Preheat the oven to 190°C (375°F) Gas 5.

Start by combining the oatmeal/oats, adding salt to taste, with the boiling water in a small saucepan. Simmer over a medium-low heat for about 10 minutes, until all the water has been absorbed (this will take less time than usual, because you're using less water).

Meanwhile, in a large frying pan/skillet or pan, melt a knob of butter (or a splash of olive oil) – enough to cover the base of the pan – over a medium-high heat. Add the mushrooms and a pinch of salt and sauté for 3–5 minutes until seared and releasing water. Remove from the heat.

Stir the mushrooms and their juices, along with half of the thyme leaves, into the cooked oatmeal/oats. Add this mixture to the greased frying pan/skillet or baking dish, spreading evenly. Dot with ricotta and sprinkle with the remaining thyme leaves. Make two hollows in the mixture and crack the eggs into them.

Bake in the preheated oven for 10–15 minutes until the egg whites are just set. Serve warm (taking care with the hot pan handle), adding more salt and some black pepper to taste.

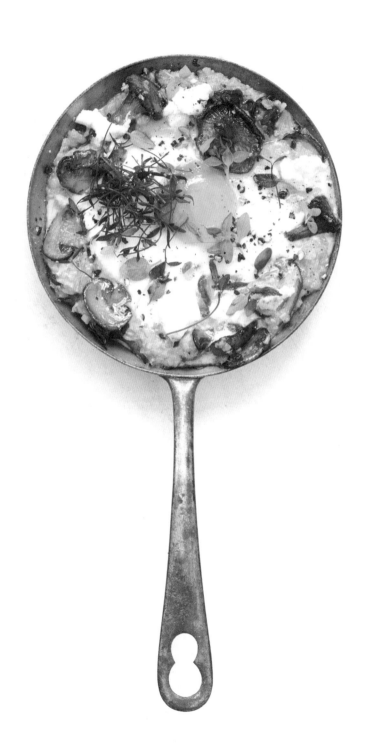

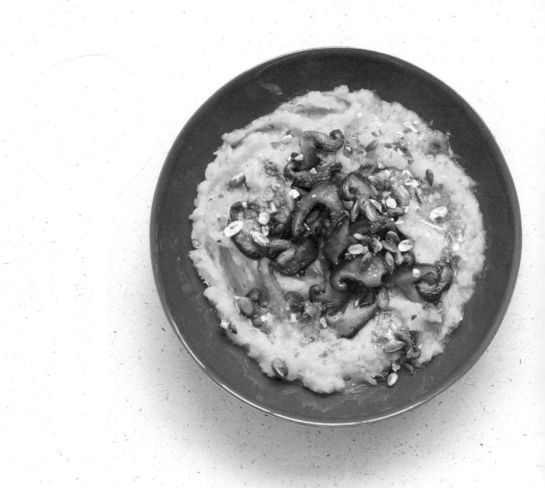

# BUTTERNUT PURÉE PORRIDGE

SIMILAR TO THE SWEET POTATO PURÉE PORRIDGE ON PAGE 80, THIS
IS A FRIENDLY VEGETABLE MASH THAT'S BEEN BUMPED TO PORRIDGE
STATUS WITH A FEW PUNCHY TOPPINGS. USING THE HERB BUTTER
(FROM PAGE 139) ADDS THE PERFECT SAVOURY NOTE.

**500 ml/2 cups water or stock
of choice**

**1 kg/2 lb. butternut squash, peeled,
seeded and cut into cubes**

**2 tablespoons Herb Butter (page 139)
or grass-fed butter**

**sea salt, to taste**

**OPTIONAL TOPPINGS**

**75 g/½ cup Shiitake Mushroom
'Bacon' (page 45), to serve**

**toasted pumpkin seeds/pepitas,
to serve**

SERVES 2

Bring the water or stock to the boil in a medium
saucepan. Add the butternut squash and a generous
pinch of salt, reduce to a simmer and cook, covered,
for 10–12 minutes, until tender.

Using a fork, potato masher or a stick blender, mash
or purée the butternut squash until smooth-ish (I find
a fork works pretty well, but it's up to you). Taste
for seasoning. Stir in the herb butter or butter and
remove from the heat.

Portion the butternut porridge into bowls. Top with
the shiitake mushroom 'bacon' and toasted pumpkin
seeds/pepitas and serve.

# BARLEY PORRIDGE WITH BRUSSELS SPROUTS

PEARL BARLEY IS ONE OF THE LONGER-COOKING GRAINS AND IT
CONTAINS GLUTEN. IF YOU'D LIKE TO SKIP IT, REPLACE IT WITH COARSE
OATMEAL/STEEL-CUT OATS OR A COMBO AS SEEN IN THE PORRIDGE
ON PAGE 116. THE OPTIONAL HERB OIL IS A BEAUTIFUL FINISHING OIL THAT
ADDS A LOT OF FLAVOUR WITH A SMALL SPOONFUL. IT'S SIMPLE TO
PREPARE, BUT IT TAKES A FEW DAYS. A REALLY NICE EXTRA VIRGIN OLIVE
OIL AND A FEW GRINDS OF PEPPER TO FINISH WOULD BE EQUALLY NICE.

185 g/1 cup pearl barley

1 litre/4 cups stock of choice

1 garlic clove, skin on and crushed
with the flat part of a chef's knife

1 tablespoon avocado or olive oil

225 g/8 oz. Brussels sprouts, woody
bases and outer leaves removed, then
thinly sliced (see Note)

salt, to taste

30 g/¼ cup crumbled blue cheese,
plus extra as desired, to serve

**OPTIONAL HERB OIL**

120 ml/½ cup extra virgin olive oil

3 sprigs of thyme

2 sprigs of rosemary

SERVES 3–4

To make the herb oil, start 4–5 days ahead. Combine
the ingredients in a screw-top glass jar, ensuring the
herbs are completely covered in oil. Store in a cool,
dark place for 4–5 days. Strain the herbs out and store
the oil in a sterilized glass jar for several months.

In a medium saucepan, combine the pearl barley,
stock, garlic and a little salt and bring to the boil over
a medium-high heat. Reduce the heat to medium-low
and simmer for 45 minutes, stirring occasionally, until
creamy and most of the liquid has been absorbed.
Remove the garlic clove and skin.

Heat the avocado or olive oil in a large frying pan/
skillet or a pan with high sides over a medium-high
heat. Add the shredded Brussels sprouts and sprinkle
with a good pinch of salt. Cook, stirring a few times,
for about 5 minutes until the Brussels sprouts are
softened, golden in places, and mostly bright green.

Portion the pearl barley into bowls and serve topped
with Brussels sprouts, crumbled blue cheese, and
a small drizzle of herb oil (if using).

**Note:** you want the Brussels sprouts to be
shredded into little ribbons. You can also do this with
a mandoline slicer – just watch your fingers!

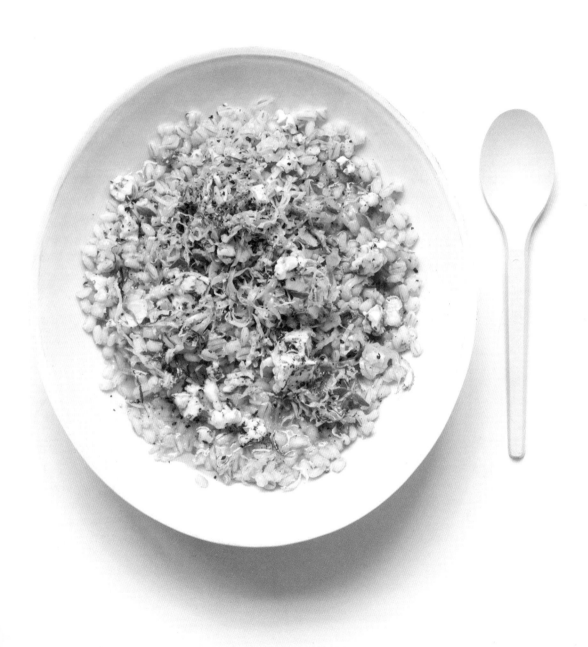

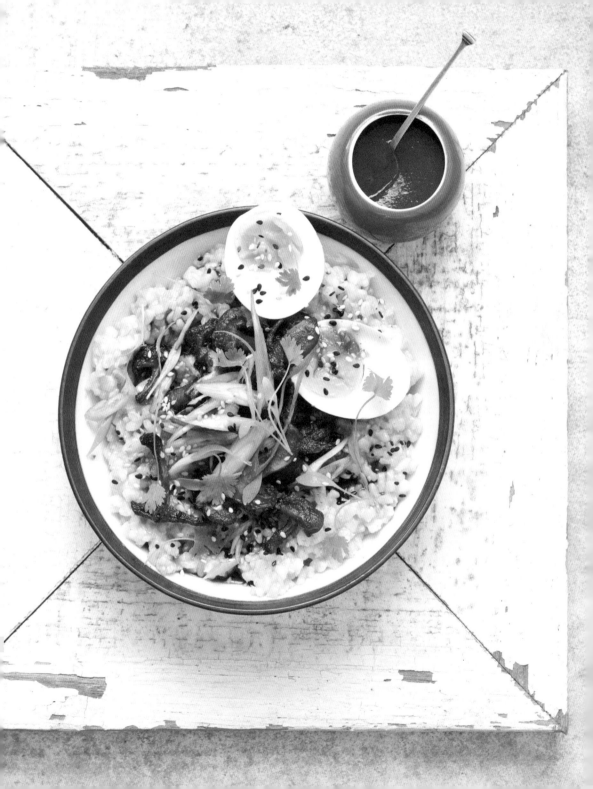

# RICE PORRIDGE

INSPIRED BY CONGEE, THIS RICE-BASED PORRIDGE USES A FEW ASIAN-STYLE TOPPINGS AND MAKES FOR A SATISFYING UMAMI-FILLED BOWL.

**200 g/1 cup short-grain brown rice**

**1 litre/4 cups stock of choice**

**2–3 eggs (1 egg per person)**

**salt, to taste**

**TO SERVE**

**splash of tamari, soy sauce or coconut aminos**

**1 quantity Shiitake Mushroom 'Bacon' (page 45)**

**2 spring onions/scallions, thinly sliced**

**2 tablespoons freshly chopped coriander/cilantro**

**sprinkling of black sesame seeds**

**sriracha sauce**

SERVES 2–3

Combine the rice and stock, with a couple of pinches of salt, in a medium saucepan. Bring to the boil, then cover with the lid slightly ajar, reduce to a simmer and cook, stirring occasionally, for 35–40 minutes. Once the rice is tender and the mixture is loose, but not too soupy, turn off the heat and leave to stand for 5 minutes. Adjust the seasoning to taste.

Meanwhile, cook medium-boiled eggs. Fill a medium saucepan two-thirds of the way full with water and bring to the boil. Once boiling, using a spoon, carefully slip the eggs into the water one at a time. Cover the saucepan with a tight-fitting lid and turn the heat off. Let stand for 7 minutes, then drain the water and transfer the eggs to a bowl filled with iced water. Once cooled, peel and slice in half lengthwise.

Portion the rice porridge into bowls and add two egg halves per bowl. Top with a splash of tamari, soy sauce or coconut aminos, shiitake mushroom 'bacon', spring onions/scallions, coriander/cilantro, sesame seeds and sriracha sauce to taste and serve.

# QUINOA AND RED LENTIL RISOTTO WITH ASPARAGUS AND PEAS

THE PAIRING OF RED LENTILS AND QUINOA IS PERFECT FOR A PLANT-BASED PROTEIN-PACKED RISOTTO. THE LENTILS COOK QUICKLY AND LOSE THEIR SHAPE, ADDING TO THE CREAMINESS OF THE DISH, WHILE QUINOA PROVIDES A PLEASANTLY NUTTY FLAVOUR AND BITE. QUICK AND LOW-MAINTENANCE, THIS IS ALSO A CHEAT'S RISOTTO WITH LESS LADLING AND STIRRING THAN TRADITIONAL VERSIONS.

## RISOTTO

**90 g/½ cup dried red lentils, soaked, then drained and rinsed**

**85 g/½ cup quinoa, soaked, then drained and rinsed**

**875 ml/3½ cups stock of choice**

**2 tablespoons finely grated Parmesan (optional), plus extra to serve**

## ASPARAGUS AND PEAS

**½ bunch asparagus (about 225 g/ 8 oz.), woody ends trimmed and cut into 2.5-cm/1-inch pieces**

**1 garlic clove, finely chopped**

**75 g/½ cup frozen peas, thawed**

**squeeze of fresh lemon juice**

**salt and freshly ground black pepper**

**olive oil or grass-fed butter, for frying**

SERVES 2

Combine the lentils, quinoa, stock and salt to taste in a medium saucepan. Cover and bring to the boil over a medium-high heat. Reduce to a simmer and cook, covered, for 15 minutes, stirring occasionally. Remove the lid and cook for another 3–5 minutes. Take off the heat when most of the liquid has been absorbed, the red lentils have broken down, and the texture is creamy. Stir in the Parmesan (if using), then taste for seasoning.

Meanwhile, heat a frying pan/skillet over a medium heat. Add enough olive oil or butter to cover the base of the pan in a thin layer and heat through for 30 seconds–1 minute. Add the asparagus, sprinkle with a generous pinch of salt and cook, stirring once or twice, for 4–5 minutes until the asparagus is browning in spots but still bright green. Add the garlic and 2 or 3 tablespoons of water if the pan is dry, and toss to combine. Cover and cook for another 1 minute. Remove the lid and stir in the peas, then remove from the heat and adjust the seasoning with salt and pepper. Add the lemon juice just before serving.

Serve the risotto topped with the asparagus and peas and more Parmesan, if desired.

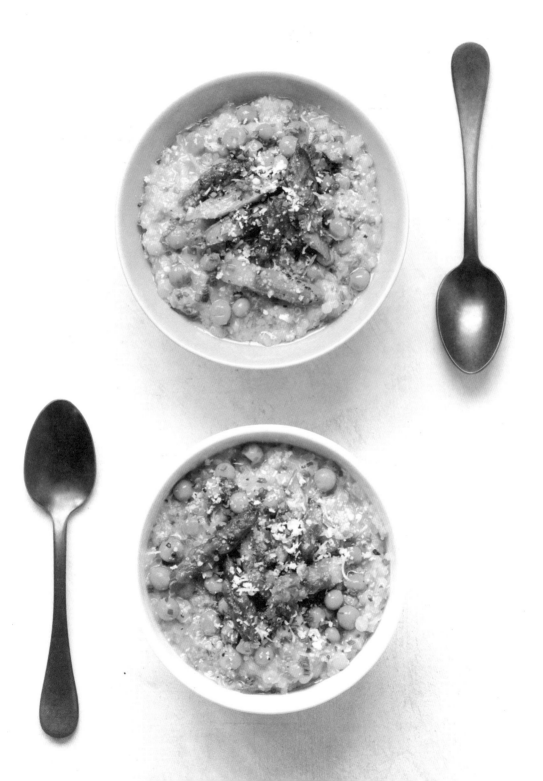

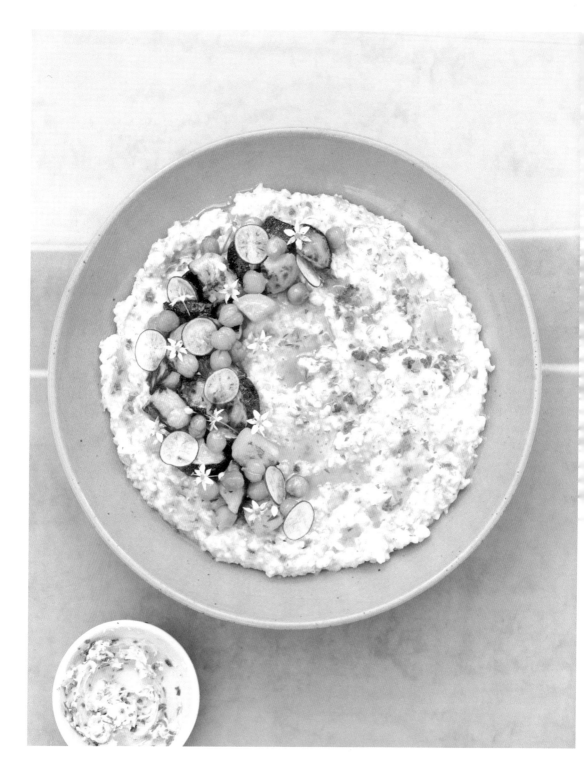

# PORRIDGE WITH ROASTED COURGETTE, CHICKPEAS AND HERB BUTTER

THE HERB BUTTER IS THE STAR OF THIS SHOW. YOU'LL HAVE SOME LEFT OVER, SO YOU CAN TRY IT WITH THE BUTTERNUT PURÉE PORRIDGE ON PAGE 131, OR SLATHERED ON TOAST AND TOPPED WITH FRESH TOMATO.

**140 g/1 cup coarse oatmeal/steel-cut oats, soaked then drained**

**1 litre/4 cups water or stock of choice**

**1 medium courgette/zucchini, chopped into 2.5-cm/1-inch pieces**

**2 teaspoons olive oil**

**140 g/1 cup cooked chickpeas, drained and dried**

**sea salt, to taste**

**HERB BUTTER**
**3 tablespoons butter, softened**

**1½ teaspoons fresh parsley, finely chopped**

**1 teaspoon chives or thyme, finely chopped**

**1 garlic clove, finely chopped**

**OPTIONAL TOPPINGS**
**1–2 small red radishes, very thinly sliced**

**edible chive flowers**

*baking sheet lined with baking parchment*

For the herb butter, in a small mixing bowl, combine the softened butter with the chopped herbs and garlic and mix well. Transfer to a ramekin and pop in the refrigerator to let the flavours mingle (you can do this step ahead).

Preheat the oven to 200°C (400°F) Gas 6.

In a medium saucepan, combine the oatmeal/oats, water or stock and a generous pinch of salt and bring to the boil over a medium-high heat. Reduce to a simmer and cook, stirring regularly, for 30 minutes.

Meanwhile, toss the courgette/zucchini with 1 teaspoon of the olive oil and a generous pinch of salt until well coated, then spread out over one half of the lined baking sheet in an even layer. Repeat with the chickpeas and remaining oil, placing them on the other ha nutes until everything is golden.

Once the porridge is cooked, portion it into bowls, swirl in a small knob of herb butter and top with the roasted courgette/zucchini and chickpeas. Scatter the radishes on top and sprinkle with a pinch of sea salt, if you like.

SERVES 2

# SUGGESTED PAIRINGS

WHY NOT CREATE YOUR OWN DELICIOUS AND NOURISHING BOWLS
BY COMBINING MY RECIPES WITH YOUR OWN FAVOURITE SIMPLE FOODS?
HERE ARE SOME DELICIOUS PAIRING IDEAS TO GET YOU STARTED.

**SWEET**

| BASE | FRUIT | TEXTURE | PROTEIN/RICHNESS |
|---|---|---|---|
| Farro | Roasted Peaches (page 34) | Hemp Seeds | Sunflower Seed Butter (page 25) |
| Mixed Oatmeal | Fresh Raspberries | Cacao Nibs | Peanut Butter |
| Buckwheat | Blueberry Compote (page 33) | Toasted Coconut Flakes (page 29) | Cashew Butter (page 26) |
| Millet | Fresh Figs | Cardamom Tahini Granola (page 38) | Honey |
| Sweet Potato | Cinnamon Apples (page 64) | Toasted Walnuts (page 30) | Tahini |
| Quinoa or Amaranth | Sliced Fresh Banana | Chocolate & Coconut Granola (page 37) | Hazelnut Butter (page 26) |
| Bircher Muesli | Berry Compote (page 33) | Toasted Pumpkin seeds/ Pepitas & Sunflower Seeds (page 30) | Greek Yogurt |

**SAVOURY**

| BASE | VEGETABLE | TEXTURE | PROTEIN/RICHNESS |
|---|---|---|---|
| Polenta | Sautéed Asparagus | Toasted Pine Nuts (page 30) | Herb Butter (page 139) |
| Oats | Roasted Cherry Tomatoes | Dukkah (page 30) | Soft-boiled Egg |
| Quinoa & Lentil Mix | Roasted Butternut Squash Cubes | Toasted Pumpkin Seeds/ Pepitas (page 30) | Herb Oil |
| Millet | Sautéed Mushrooms (page 128) | Finely Sliced Radicchio | Grated Parmesan or Nutritional Yeast Flakes |
| Farro | Red Pesto (page 42) | Microgreens or Sprouts | Crumbled Feta |

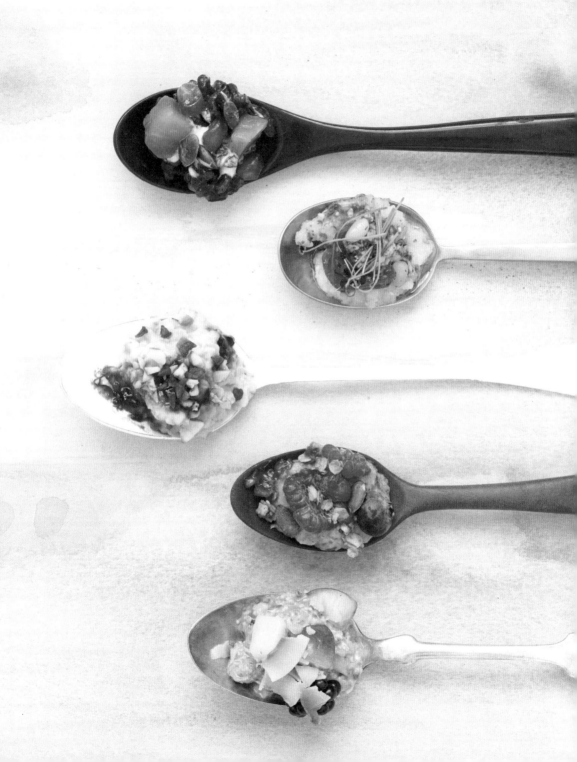

# INDEX

## ACKNOWLEDGEMENTS

A big thank you to Cindy Richards, Julia Charles and Alice Sambrook
for making this book happen. Thank you to Sharon Bowers for being in
my corner and giving me reliably great advice. To designer Sonya Nathoo,
food stylist Emily Kydd, prop stylist Alexander Breeze and photographer
Clare Winfield for making porridge look better than I could have imagined.

And to Fabian, who has my back in everything I do – even making five
batches of porridge a day in the middle of summer. I love you.

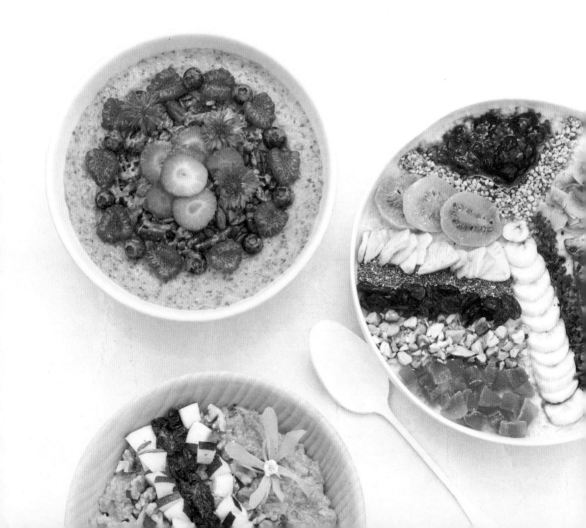

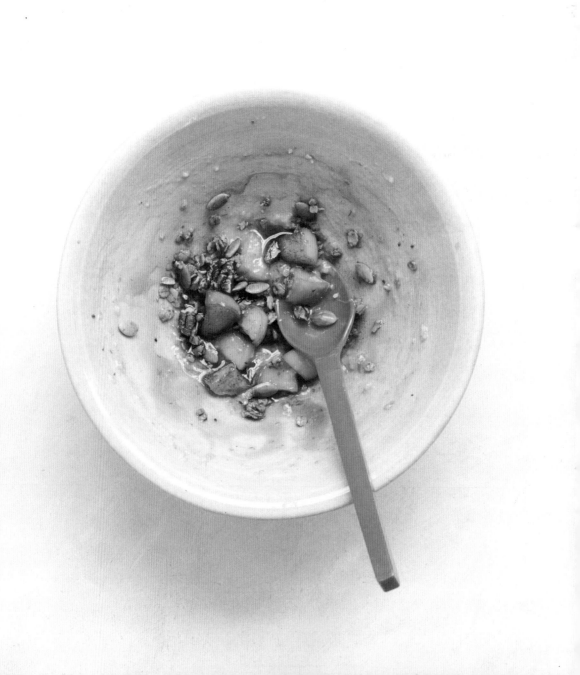